Orthopaedic Basic Sciences Postgraduate Examination

Practice MCQs and EMQs

Sebastian Dawson-Bowling

Iain McNamara

Ben Ollivere

Foreword by

Professor TWR Briggs

Orthopaedic Research UK Publishing

Orthopaedic Basic Science for the Postgraduate Examination

Orthopaedic Basic Science for the Postgraduate Examination

Practice MCQs and EMQs

Authors

Sebastian Dawson-Bowling

MA, MSc, LLM, FRCS (Tr & Orth)

Iain McNamara

MA (Cantab), MRCP, FRCS (Tr & Orth), MD

Ben Ollivere

MA (Oxon), FRCS (Tr & Orth), MD

Foreword by

Professor TWR Briggs

MD (Res), MCh (Orth), FRCS (Ed), FRCS (Eng)

Managing editor

Arash Angadji

BEng (Hons), MSc, PhD, MBA

First published in Great Britain in 2012 by
Orthopaedic Research UK Publishing

ISBN 978-0-9573469-0-1

Cover design: Chacha
Indexer: Laurence Errington

Produced by
The Choir Press, Gloucester

Contents

Foreword

One of the key challenges confronting candidates preparing for post-graduate examinations in trauma and orthopaedics is that of striking a balance – between on the one hand acquiring the general overview required for a broad understanding of the subject, whilst on the other memorising the detailed minutiae that will be tested in all parts of the examination, but in particular in the written section. Another problem faced is that, of the many outstanding textbooks currently available, relatively few focus specifically on the orthopaedic basic sciences, despite the substantial proportion of the examination allocated to this area of the curriculum.

This excellent book has been developed simultaneously to address both these issues. It would be impossible to encompass every aspect of the basic science syllabus in a text of this size and format; however, over more than 500 questions the authors have successfully covered all the key areas likely to be encountered in the FRCS (Tr & Orth) or equivalent, including anatomy and surgical approaches. Each chapter comprises both single best answer and extended matching sections, followed by detailed explanations of all correct and incorrect responses. The extensive index allows easy access to key topics and enhances the book's value as a reference text.

The authors are all approaching, or have achieved completion of higher surgical and fellowship training, whilst having sufficiently recent experience of postgraduate orthopaedic examinations to ensure that the questions are representative of the level and scope required. Furthermore, all three have regularly taught on the hugely successful Orthopaedic Research UK revision courses.

Drawing partly on material from these courses, the book simultaneously provides a tool for assessing knowledge levels and a means of rapidly assimilating detailed facts. The authors and the team at Orthopaedic

Research UK are to be commended on a highly successful collaboration. Having studied the text carefully, I am confident that it will form a central part of the examination candidate's armoury for many years to come.

Professor Tim W R Briggs MD (Res), MCh (Orth), FRCS (Ed), FRCS (Eng)
Consultant Orthopaedic Surgeon and Joint Head of Training,
Royal National Orthopaedic Hospital, Stanmore;
Vice President and President Elect, British Orthopaedic Association

Preface

Gaining knowledge and experience in orthopaedics, sufficient to pass the requisite examinations, is a daunting task and any extra help is to be welcomed.

Three young, successful orthopaedic surgeons have decided to pass on their recently acquired knowledge of basic sciences and enthusiastically devoted hours of work to compiling this book. Despite being on opposite sides of the globe they have managed to put together a volume which will test and educate the student/trainee in a format which reflects the FRCS (Tr & Orth) examination.

Orthopaedic Research UK is an independent charity dedicated to advancing orthopaedic knowledge, not just by funding and publishing cutting-edge research, but also by organising surgeon training and education.

We were, therefore, delighted to collaborate in the publishing of this work. All proceeds from sales will, of course, be invested back into orthopaedic research.

We hope the contents and format of this book will help you not only to pass the exam, but to build the basis of a successful career in orthopaedics.

Brian Jones
Chief Executive
Orthopaedic Research UK

Acknowledgments

We are very grateful to the invaluable contribution of Orthopaedic Research UK to the conception and publication of this book. Especially we would like to thank Brian Jones and Arash Angadji for their support throughout the whole project.

We would also like to thank the various trainers and mentors, past and present, who have advised, guided and supported us through all aspects of our careers so far.

On a more personal note:

I would sincerely like to thank my wife, Emma, who must feel like a single mother much of the time, and our children Elspeth and Daniel, for all their love and support throughout this and my endless other projects. – SJDB

I would like to thank my wife, Kate, and daughter, Tessa, for their remarkable support and understanding through all of our (ad)ventures. – IRM

I would like to especially thank the two Katies in my life for help, understanding, endless patience and mostly tolerance with my questionable 'work/life' balance. – BJO

May 2012

Chapter 1
Anatomy and Surgical Approaches

MCQ 35
EMQ 10

Multiple Choice Questions

1. **Which one of the following correctly describes the contents of the IVth extensor compartment of the wrist?**
    a. Extensor indicis proprius, extensor digiti minimi
    b. Extensor digitorum communis, extensor pollicis longus
    c. Extensor pollicis longus
    d. Extensor digitorum communis, extensor indicis proprius
    e. Extensor indicis proprius, extensor pollicis longus

2. **During the initial stages of the Smith-Peterson approach to the hip, an internervous plane is developed between the sartorius and tensor fasciae latae. As these are retracted, which one of the following structures traverses the operative field, overlying the rectus femoris muscle?**
    a. Obturator branch of the femoral nerve
    b. Ascending branch of lateral femoral circumflex artery
    c. Lateral cutaneous nerve of the thigh
    d. Descending branch of medial femoral circumflex artery
    e. Ascending branch of medial femoral circumflex artery

3. **The nerve supply to the pectoralis minor muscle is derived from:**

   a. The lower trunk of the brachial plexus

   b. The ansa cervicalis

   c. The posterior cord of the brachial plexus

   d. Both the medial and posterior cords of the brachial plexus

   e. Both the medial and lateral cords of the brachial plexus

4. **The anterior interosseous nerve:**

   a. Forms the terminal motor branch of the radial nerve in the forearm

   b. Arises from the median nerve below pronator teres to supply flexor pollicis longus, pronator quadratus and the lateral half of flexor digitorum profundus

   c. Arises from the median nerve below supinator to supply flexor carpi radialis, palmaris longus and the medial half of flexor digitorum superficialis

   d. Forms the terminal sensory branch of the radial nerve in the forearm

   e. Arises from the median nerve below pronator teres to supply flexorpollicis longus, pronator quadratus and the medial half of flexor digitorum profundus

5. **The anterior tibial artery:**

   a. Supplies the main direct arterial (nutrient) supply to the tibia

   b. Supplies the main arterial supply to the peroneus brevis muscle

   c. Continues into the foot as the medial plantar artery

   d. Commences at the popliteal trifurcation, passing between the heads of gastrocnemius before winding round the medial border of the tibia to enter the anterior compartment

   e. Commences at popliteal trifurcation, passing between the heads of tibialis posterior before crossing the interosseous membrane into the anterior compartment

6. **The sciatic nerve:**

    a. Provides the main sensory supply to the buttock

    b. Is formed in the upper sacral plexus from the anterior primary rami of L3, L4, L5, S1 and S2

    c. Exits the pelvis via the lesser sciatic foramen where it is closely related to the piriformis and short external rotators

    d. Supplies sensation to all skin distal to the knee

    e. Normally divides into the popliteal and common peroneal nerves approximately two-thirds of the way down the thigh

7. **During the posterior approach to the hip:**

    a. The fibres of gluteus medius are split following incision of the fascia lata, allowing visualisation of the piriformis and short external rotators

    b. Formal repair of the posterior structures, although commonly undertaken, has been shown to confer no reduction in the risk of dislocation

    c. The piriformis, gemelli and obturator internus are detached from the greater trochanter allowing exposure of the underlying capsule

    d. Extension of the approach distally is less easily undertaken than with the modified Hardinge (lateral) approach

    e. The posterior capsule and short rotators are visualised more readily if the assistant externally rotates the hip

8. **During the posterior approach to the shoulder:**

    a. The scapular portion of the deltoid origin is detached in its entirety from the spine of the scapula

    b. The internervous plane between the axillary and infrascapular nerves is utilised

    c. Axillary nerve injury is less likely than with the deltopectoral approach

    d. The joint capsule is visualised by inferior retraction of teres major

    e. The trunks of the brachial plexus should always be formally visualised to reduce the risk of iatrogenic damage

9   During the anterior approach to the cervical spine, a plane is developed between the anterior border of sternocleidomastoid and the posterior borders of the sternohyoid and sternothyroid, allowing visualisation of the carotid sheath. However, subsequent development of the interval between the sheath and the midline structures may be limited by two arteries passing across this plane. What is the identity of these two vessels?

   a. Ascending cervical and inferior laryngeal arteries
   b. Superficial cervical and ascending pharyngeal arteries
   c. Superior and inferior laryngeal arteries
   d. Superior and inferior thyroid arteries
   e. Thyroidea ima and cricothyroid arteries

10 Hunter's canal (adductor canal of the thigh):

   a. Is the normal site of division of the sciatic nerve into its terminal tibial and common peroneal branches
   b. Is bounded medially by adductors longus and magnus, laterally by vastus medialis, with a fascial roof covered by sartorius
   c. Is bounded medially by adductors longus and brevis, and laterally by the adductor portion of adductor magnus
   d. Contains the femoral nerve and vessels
   e. Is bounded medially by adductors longus and magnus, laterally by vastus intermedius, with a fascial roof covered by sartorius

11. Which one of the following statements about the medial collateral ligament (MCL) of the elbow is TRUE?

   a. The posterior bundle is fully taut between full extension and 60° of flexion
   b. The MCL is formed of the ulnar collateral ligament, the lateral ulnar collateral ligament and Cooper's transverse bundle
   c. The MCL is formed of the ulnar collateral ligament, the lateral ulnar collateral ligament and Cooper's transverse bundle
   d. The anterior bundle (ulnar collateral ligament) is the most important ligamentous structure in withstanding valgus stressing of the elbow
   e. The anterior bundle (ulnar collateral ligament) is fully taut between full extension and 60° of flexion

12. The deltoid ligament of the ankle is formed of:

a. The tibionavicular, tibiocalcaneal, anterior tibiotalar and posterior tibiotalar ligaments

b. The anterior tibiofibular, posterior tibiofibular, tibionavicular and tibiocalcaneal ligaments

c. The talonavicular, talocalcaneal, tibionavicular and tibiocalcaneal ligaments

d. The fibulocuboid, calcaneofibular, anterior tibiofibular and posterior tibiofibular ligaments

e. The tibionavicular, tibiocalcaneal, fibulocuboid and talocalcaneal ligaments

13. The ilioinguinal approach:

a. Makes use of the internervous plane between the obturator and femoral nerves

b. Makes use of the internervous plane between the femoral and superior gluteal nerves

c. Is characterised by the creation of three 'windows' defined from lateral to medial by the iliopsoas tendon and iliac vessels respectively

d. Does not allow visualisation of the sacro-iliac joint

e. May be used in combination with a Stoppa approach

14. The quadrangular space of the shoulder is bounded by:

a. Teres major inferiorly, teres minor superiorly, the long head of triceps laterally and the circumflex scapular artery medially

b. Teres major superiorly, the long head of triceps medially, the lateral head of triceps laterally and the radial nerve and profunda brachii inferiorly

c. Subscapularis and teres minor superiorly, teres major inferiorly, the long head of triceps medially and the humeral shaft laterally

d. Pectoralis major and minor anteriorly, subscapularis posteriorly, serratus anterior medially and coracobrachialis and biceps laterally

e. Teres major inferiorly, the long head of triceps medially, the humeral shaft laterally and the inferior glenohumeral ligament superiorly

15. During the posterior approach to the humerus:

a. The long head of the triceps is retracted laterally and the medial head medially, to expose the underlying lateral head

b. The radial nerve can be clearly visualised in the spiral groove which separates the lateral head of the triceps from the coraco-brachialis insertion

c. The long head of the triceps is retracted medially and the lateral head laterally, to expose the deeper medial head lying immediately distal and medial to the spiral groove

d. An internervous plane is utilised between the radial and musculocutaneous nerves

e. An internervous plane is utilised between the radial and axillary nerves

16. In the knee, the ligament of Wrisberg:

a. Arises from the posterior horn of the lateral meniscus, running anteriorly to the PCL to insert into the lateral aspect of the medial femoral condyle

b. May be confused with the PCL at arthroscopy

c. Together with the biceps tendon forms the middle of Seebacher's three layers of the lateral side of the knee

d. Is believed to have a role as a secondary restraint to posterior tibial translation following posterior cruciate ligament rupture

e. Is thought frequently to be damaged at the same time as a twisting injury to the posterior horn of the medial meniscus

17. The medial (Ludloff) approach to the hip:

a. Utilises the internervous plane between the obturator and inferior gluteal nerves

b. Utilises two intermuscular planes; the first between gracilis and adductor longus; the second, deeper plane between adductor brevis and adductor magnus

c. Utilises two intermuscular planes; the first between sartorius and gracilis; the second, deeper plane between the two portions of adductor magnus

d. Utilises the internervous plane between the medial and lateral branches of the obturator nerve

e. Has been shown to be associated with a 5% risk of injury to the nerve to obturator internus

18. **Which of the following is found in the third plantar layer of the foot?**
    a. Quadratus plantae muscle
    b. Flexor hallucis brevis muscle
    c. Flexor digitorum brevis muscle
    d. Peroneus longus tendon
    e. Tibialis posterior tendon

19. **Which of the following provides the primary static restraint to inferior translation of the humeral head when the shoulder is abducted to 90°?**
    a. Superior glenohumeral ligament
    b. Middle glenohumeral ligament
    c. Inferior glenohumeral ligament
    d. Coracohumeral ligament
    e. Long head of biceps

20. **The sustentaculum tali:**
    a. Contains the tibial nerve and posterior tibial artery
    b. Is an eminence situated on the anterolateral aspect of the os calcis
    c. Is an eminence situated on the anteroinferior aspect of the talus
    d. Is an eminence situated on the posteroinferior aspect of the talus
    e. Has a groove on its inferior surface through which passes the flexor hallucis longus tendon

21. **Which of the following statements, concerning the surgical anatomy of the popliteal fossa encountered during the posterior approach to the knee, is TRUE?**
    a. As the small saphenous vein pierces the popliteal fascia it lies lateral to the sural nerve
    b. The popliteal artery lies superficial to the popliteal vein but deep to the tibial nerve
    c. When the knee is extended the medial and lateral middle genicular arteries arise from the popliteal artery at the level of the tibial plateau
    d. The common peroneal nerve usually divides into its terminal deep and superficial branches within the substance of peroneus longus
    e. The popliteal artery lies lateral to the popliteal vein as it enters the fossa from above, but crosses to lie medial to the vein as it continues into the calf

22. **Posterior access to the first two cervical vertebrae may be achieved via dissection of the suboccipital triangle. Which two neurovascular structures are most likely to be at potential risk during this approach?**
    a. The occipital artery and the great occipital nerve
    b. The occipital artery and the lesser occipital nerve
    c. The vertebral artery and the great occipital nerve
    d. The vertebral artery and the lesser occipital nerve
    e. The vertebral vein and the lesser occipital nerve

23. **With of the following statements concerning the flexor digitorum profundus is TRUE?**
    a. It originates from the anterior shaft of the radius and adjoining interosseous membrane
    b. The tendon to the index finger separates more proximally than those to the remaining three fingers
    c. In the fingers each of the four tendons divides into two slips which insert into the sides of the middle phalanx
    d. In addition to finger flexion there is a secondary role as a weak supinator of the forearm
    e. The medial half of the muscle is innervated by the anterior interosseous branch of the median nerve

24. **During the posterolateral approach to the ankle:**
    a. An internervous plane is developed between the superficial and deep peroneal nerves
    b. Peroneus longus is identifiable by the fact that it remains muscular almost to the ankle, whilst peroneus brevis is tendinous at this level
    c. Flexor hallucis longus is identifiable as a muscular structure arising from the posteromedial aspect of the distal fibula and interosseous membrane
    d. Peroneus tertius should be retracted laterally to protect the short saphenous vein and sural nerve
    e. It is sometimes necessary to detach tibialis posterior from its fibular origin to obtain adequate exposure of the ankle join

25. **Which of the following best describes the osteology of the distal humerus in males?**
    a. 4° valgus, 20° anterior angulation
    b. 7° valgus, 20° anterior angulation
    c. 7° valgus, 30° anterior angulation
    d. 10° valgus, 20° anterior angulation
    e. 12° valgus, 30° anterior angulation

26. **The uncovertebral joints of Luschka:**
    a. Are present throughout the cervical, thoracic and lumbar spine
    b. Are present only between the 7 cervical vertebrae
    c. Lie immediately medial to the vertebral arteries
    d. Are stabilised by the anterior longitudinal ligament
    e. Are stabilised by the posterior longitudinal ligament

27. **Within the spinal cord, the dorsal column transmits:**
    a. Ipsilateral sensation to vibration, light touch and proprioception
    b. Contralateral sensation to vibration, light touch and proprioception
    c. Contralateral motor function
    d. Ipsilateral motor function
    e. Ipsilateral sensation to pain and temperature

28. **A 29-year-old man working with industrial machinery develops compartment syndrome in his lower leg after a crush injury. He is taken to theatre for urgent fasciotomy via a two incision approach. Part of this technique:**
    a. Allows the anterior and deep posterior compartments to be decompressed through a single anterior incision midway between the fibula and tibia
    b. Allows the deep posterior and medial compartments to be decompressed through a single medial incision 2 cm posterior to the palpable posteromedial edge of the tibia
    c. Allows the anterior and medial compartments to be decompressed through a single medial incision 2 cm anterior to the palpable posteromedial edge of the tibia
    d. Allows the lateral and anterior compartments to be decompressed through a single incision 2 cm anterior to fibular shaft
    e. Allows the lateral and deep posterior compartments to be decompressed through a single incision 2 cm posterior to fibular shaft

29. **During the anterior approach to the elbow via the cubital fossa, which important structure is encountered emerging between biceps and brachialis to the lateral side of the biceps tendon?**

    a. Median nerve
    b. Brachial artery
    c. Radial nerve
    d. Lateral branch of basilic vein
    e. Lateral cutaneous nerve of forearm

30. **The femoral triangle is bounded:**

    a. Superiorly by the inguinal ligament, medially by the medial border of adductor longus and laterally by the medial border of sartorius
    b. Superiorly by the inguinal ligament, medially by the medial border of adductor magnus and laterally by the lateral border of sartorius
    c. Superiorly by the inguinal ligament, medially by the medial border of gracilis and laterally by the medial border of pectineus
    d. Superiorly by the inguinal ligament, medially by the medial border of iliacus and laterally by the medial border of sartorius
    e. Superiorly by the inguinal ligament, medially by the lateral border of adductor brevis and laterally by the lateral border of sartorius

31. **If the shoulder is accessed via the deltopectoral approach, retraction of the conjoined tendon is required to enable visualisation of the anterior joint capsule. The retractor should never be placed medial to the tendon because of the specific risk to:**

    a. The cephalic vein
    b. The lateral pectoral nerve
    c. The lower subscapular nerve
    d. The musculocutaneous nerve
    e. The lateral thoracic artery

32. A 73-year-old man presents to the orthopaedic clinic complaining of low back pain and radicular symptoms in both legs. His imaging reveals a degenerative L4/L5 spondylolisthesis. What would be the most likely findings on neurological assessment?

    a. Weak ankle dorsiflexion, reduced sensation over the dorsum of the foot and normal reflexes
    b. Normal ankle dorsiflexion but weak toe extension, reduced sensation in the dorsum of the foot and reduced patellar tendon reflex
    c. Normal ankle dorsiflexion but weak toe extension, reduced sensation in the dorsum of the foot and normal reflexes
    d. Weak eversion of the foot, reduced sensation over the lateral aspect of the foot and normal reflexes
    e. Weak eversion of the foot, reduced sensation over the lateral aspect of the foot and reduced Achilles' tendon reflex

33. The erector spinae muscle group comprises:

    a. Iliocostalis, longissimus and spinalis
    b. Iliocostalis, semispinalis and multifidus
    c. Longissimus, spinalis and semispinalis
    d. Quadratus lumborum, interspinalis and splenius capitis
    e. Semispinalis, multifidus and rotatores

34. A firefighter overbalances off the edge of a balcony but is saved from dropping four floors when his colleague catches him by the left upper limb as he falls. He subsequently presents to hospital complaining of weakness in the affected limb. Examination of his face is normal. Clinically, the limb is noted to be held in an internally rotated position, with the elbow extended, the forearm pronated and the wrist and fingers flexed. What is the most likely diagnosis?

    a. Avulsion of suprascapular nerve
    b. Pre-ganglionic upper brachial plexus injury
    c. Pre-ganglionic lower brachial plexus injury
    d. Post-ganglionic upper brachial plexus injury
    e. Post-ganglionic lower brachial plexus injury

35. The natatory ligament:

a. Passes along the side of the finger separating Cleland's ligaments from the digital vessels

b. Resists excessive abduction of the fingers

c. Crosses the web spaces deep to the spiral bands but superficial to the digital vessels

d. Crosses the web spaces superficial to the spiral bands but deep to the digital vessels

e. Is crossed volarly by the four lumbricals

Extended Matching Questions

SCENARIO I OPTIONS

A Conoid ligament
B Trapezoid ligament
C Short head of biceps
D Long head of biceps
E Long head of triceps

F Rhomboid major
G Levator scapulae
H Infrascapular nerve
I Suprascapular nerve
J Upper subscapular nerve

This question concerns anatomical structures relating to the scapula. For each stem below, choose the SINGLE correct anatomical structure from the list of options. Each option may be used once, more than once, or not at all.

1. This structure arises from the upper trunk of the brachial plexus and travels laterally under omohyoid and trapezius to pass under the superior transverse scapular ligament and into the supraspinous fossa. It finally curves around the lateral border of the scapular spine to enter the infraspinous fossa.

2. Originating from the coracoid process, this is the most medial of the structures stabilising the distal clavicle; significant acromioclavicular joint disruption implies complete disruption of this structure.

3. This structure is a depressor and secondary stabiliser of the glenohumeral joint.

4. This muscle has an action in retraction of the scapula. Its point of attachment is along the medial border of the scapula immediately behind serratus anterior. It is innervated by the dorsal scapular nerve.

5. This nerve is the first branch of the posterior cord of the brachial plexus.

SCENARIO II OPTIONS

A Medial antebrachial cutaneous nerve

B Anterior interosseous nerve

C Posterior interosseous nerve

D Median nerve

E Radial nerve

F Supinator

G Pronator teres

H Pronator quadratus

I Flexor carpi ulnaris

J Flexor carpi radialis

This question concerns the surgical anatomy of the forearm. For each stem below, choose the SINGLE correct anatomical structure from the list of options. Each option may be used once, more than once, or not at all.

6. This nerve enters the forearm by passing between the two heads of supinator.

7. This nerve enters the forearm by passing between the two heads of pronator teres.

8. This nerve lies on flexor digitorum profundus covered by flexor digitorum superficialis.

9. This muscle receives its motor innervation from the anterior interosseous nerve.

10. This muscle is the most lateral of the group originating from the common flexor origin at the medial epicondyle.

Answers: Chapter 1

MCQ 35
EMQ 10

Multiple Choice Answers

1. D A knowledge of the extensor compartments is essential to the accurate assessment of sharp injuries to the dorsum of the wrist, as well as the planning of surgical approaches. The contents of the six compartments (running from lateral to medial) are:

I – Abductor pollicis longus, extensor pollicis brevis

II – Extensor carpi radialis longus, extensor carpi radialis brevis

III – Extensor pollicis longus

IV – Extensor digitorum communis, extensor indicis proprius

V – Extensor digiti minimi

VI – Extensor carpi ulnaris

2. B The anterior approach to the hip utilises the internervous plane between the femoral and superior gluteal nerves. The initial dissection is between the sartorius and tensor fasciae latae muscles, at which point the ascending branch of lateral femoral circumflex artery must be identified and may need to be ligated. The dissection then continues in the same plane, between the rectus femoris and gluteus medius; to expose the hip capsule. The straight and reflected heads of the rectus may then be detached respectively from the anterior inferior iliac spine and the front of the hip capsule and the ilium immediately above to improve exposure. There is no obturator branch of the femoral nerve.

3. E The orthopaedic surgeon must have a detailed knowledge of the roots, trunks, divisions and cords that comprise the brachial plexus. Pectoralis minor, like pectoralis major, receives a dual innervation from both the lateral pectoral nerve (arising directly from the lateral cord) and the medial pectoral nerve (from the medial cord) (although some sources do state only the medial pectoral nerve). The ansa cervicalis is found in the neck, supplying the strap muscles.

4. B The median nerve gives off its anterior interosseous branch at a variable point below the two heads of pronator teres, providing motor supply to flexor pollicis longus, pronator quadratus and the radial half of flexor digitorum profundus; and may also provide sensory supply to part of the wrist and distal radioulnar joint. The terminal motor branch of the radial nerve is the posterior interosseous nerve; the terminal sensory branch is the superficial radial nerve.

5. E The anterior tibial artery commences beneath the fibrous arch of soleus, immediately distal to popliteus. After passing between the heads of tibialis posterior the artery passes medial to the fibular neck at the upper border of the interosseous membrane to enter the anterior compartment, where it supplies the extensor structures before continuing into the foot as the dorsalis pedis. The main nutrient artery to the tibia arises from the posterior tibial artery, shortly after the former gives rise to the peroneal artery, which in turn supplies both peroneus longus and brevis. The medial plantar artery is a terminal branch of the posterior tibial artery.

6. E The sciatic nerve arises from the anterior primary rami of L4, L5, S1, S2 and S3. It exits the pelvis via the greater sciatic foramen where it is closely related to the piriformis and short external rotators. Before exiting the pelvis it gives rise to the nerve to quadratus femoris and the nerve to obturator internus, which similarly exit the pelvis through the greater sciatic foramen, before between them supplying the hip joint and the majority of the short external rotators. The sciatic nerve itself gives no branches in the buttock, which receives its sensory supply from the iliohypogastric nerve and the primary posterior rami of L1, L2 and L3. Although the majority of the sensation distal to the knee is supplied by the terminal branches of the sciatic nerve, the sensory supply to the skin on the medial aspect of the lower leg is derived from the saphenous nerve, the terminal branch of the femoral nerve. Division of the sciatic to popliteal and common proneal nerve is highly variable, but commonly occurs two-thirds of the way down the thigh.

7. C The posterior approach to the hip is popular amongst arthroplasty surgeons due to the fact that it is more readily extensile than other approaches, as well as not breaching the abductor mechanism of gluteus medius, gluteus minimus and tensor fasciae latae. After splitting the fascia lata and gluteus maximus in the line of its fibres, the surgeon asks the assistant to internally rotate the leg allowing clear visualisation of the piriformis, gemelli and obturator internus as they insert into the inner surface of the greater trochanter. Pellicci *et al. (JBJS-Am 1998)* showed that formal repair of the capsule and rotators prior to closure significantly reduced the risk of dislocation post-operatively.

8. A The posterior approach to the shoulder is less commonly undertaken than the anterior and lateral approaches, but is needed at times for the treatment of some chronic dislocations or fracture disloca- tions, as well as the siting of a posterior bone block in patients with recurrent posterior instability. After detachment of the scapular origin of deltoid, an internervous plane is identified between infraspinatus (suprascapular nerve) and teres minor (axillary nerve); the latter is retracted inferiorly to expose the infero-posterior aspect of the shoulder joint. Care should be taken to avoid injury to the axillary nerve which is closely related to the teres minor muscle. No part of the brachial plexus may be visualised during this procedure.

9. D The anterior approach to the cervical spine is a surprisingly common exam question. Both the superior and inferior thyroid arteries (arising respectively from the common carotid artery and the thyrocer- vical trunk) cross the interval between the carotid sheath and the midline; both are therefore at risk during the development of this plane, depending on the precise cervical level requiring access. Rarely, ligation and division of one or other may be necessary; with the inferior thyroid artery in particular, care should be taken to avoid accidental division which may result in retraction of the vessel behind the carotid sheath, where it is difficult to access.

10. B Hunter's subsartorial (adductor) canal is bounded medially by adductors longus and magnus, and laterally by vastus medialis. Its roof is formed by fascia containing the subsartorial plexus, and the sartorius muscle overlying this. The canal contains the femoral artery and vein, along with the saphenous nerve (a terminal branch of the femoral nerve). The sciatic nerve gives rise to its terminal tibial and common peroneal branches in the posterior aspect of the thigh, normally approximately two-thirds of the way down the femur (although rarely the division has already taken place by the time the nerves exit the pelvis via the greater sciatic foramen).

11. D The MCL of the elbow arises from the medial epicondyle and is formed of three bundles; anterior (ulnar collateral ligament), posterior and transverse (Cooper's ligament). The anterior bundle has a key role in withstanding valgus stress, especially with the forearm in pronation. The posterior bundle is fan shaped and taut only to 30° of flexion. The lateral collateral ligament conversely arises from the lateral epicondyle, and is formed of the radial collateral ligament, the annular ligament and the lateral ulnar collateral ligament.

12. A The ligaments of the ankle are dense strong structures, accounting for the fact that trauma often results in bony avulsion rather than ligamentous injury (although clearly the two may also occur together). The deltoid ligament complex is sited over the medial aspect of the ankle joint, and comprises superficial and deep layers. The superficial layer is made of the tibionavicular and tibiocalcaneal ligaments; the deep layer of the anterior and posterior tibiotalar ligaments. There is no fibulocuboid ligament.

13. C The ilioinguinal approach is used both in the operative management of acetabular injuries, and during some periacetabular osteotomies. No internervous plane is utilised; the incision runs above and parallel to the inguinal ligament, subsequent to which the external oblique aponeurosis is detached from the iliac wing. The lateral femoral cutaneous nerve frequently has to be sacrificed at this stage. Once the iliacus and rectus abdominis have been stripped away from the ilium and pubis respectively, deeper dissection allows isolation of the iliopsoas tendon and iliac vessels. These are protected with rubber slings, and allow the operative field to be subdivided into windows. The lateral window allows visualisation not only of the internal iliac fossa but also of the sacro-iliac joint if necessary. The Stoppa approach is an extraperitoneal midline approach commonly used to access the inner table of the pelvis and anterior column for acetabular fracture fixation.

14. C Questions about the anatomical spaces within the axilla are common in both written and oral parts of postgraduate orthopaedic examinations. The candidate should therefore be able to describe their boundaries and contents:

- Quadrangular space – subscapularis and teres minor superiorly, teres major inferiorly, the long head of triceps medially and the humeral shaft laterally; contains axillary nerve, posterior circum-flex humeral artery and vein

- Triangular space (medial triangular space) – teres minor superiorly, teres major inferiorly, long head of triceps laterally; contains circumflex scapular artery

- Triangular interval (lateral triangular space) – teres major superiorly, the long head of triceps medially, the lateral head of triceps laterally; contains the radial nerve and profunda brachii artery

The *axilla* as a whole contains the main nerves and vessels supplying the upper limb, as well as the chief lymphatic drainage. Its boundaries are as follows:

- Anterior wall – pectoralis major and minor, subclavius, suspensory axillary ligament and the clavipectoral fascia

- Posterior wall – subscapularis, latissimus dorsi and teres major

- Base – skin and subcutaneous tissue

- Lateral wall – biceps and coracobrachialis in close relation to humerus

- Medial wall – serratus anterior and underlying ribs

- Superiorly – outer border of first rib, superior border of scapula, posterior border of clavicle

15. C The posterior approach to the humerus has the advantage of being fully extensile – if needed it can run from the surgical neck of the humerus down as far as the olecranon fossa. The approach utilises a plane between the long head of triceps medially and the lateral head laterally; this is not a true internervous plane as all three heads receive their innervation from the radial nerve. Once the plane is established the radial nerve and profunda brachii artery may be visualised lying proximal to the medial head of triceps, which lies deep to the lateral and long heads; the medial head is incised and stripped subperiosteally to expose the underlying humeral shaft. Whilst the radial nerve is identified in the spiral groove coracobrachialis is an anterior structure and not seen posteriorly.

16. **D** The anterior (Humphrey's) and posterior (Wrisberg's) meniscofemoral ligaments both originate from the posterior horn of the lateral meniscus and pass up to the lateral aspect of the medial femoral condyle. Wrisberg's ligament runs posterior to the PCL; Humphrey's ligament passes anterior to the PCL, with which it may be confused during knee arthroscopy. There is no association between medial meniscal injury and damage to these ligaments, which are related to the lateral not medial meniscus. Following complete transection of the PCL, it is thought that the two meniscofemoral ligaments together have a secondary restraining role in posterior translation of the tibia.
Seebacher's three lateral layers respectively comprise:

I. biceps tendon and iliotibial band

II. patellar retinaculum, patellofemoral ligaments

III. superficial lamina (lateral collateral and fabellofibular ligaments) and deep lamina (arcuate ligament and joint capsule), coronary ligament, popliteus, popliteofibular ligament.

17. **B** The medial approach to the hip develops two intermuscular planes; the first between gracilis and adductor longus (both supplied by the anterior branch of the obturator nerve); the second, deeper plane between adductor brevis (anterior division of the obturator nerve) and adductor magnus (whose adductor and ischial portions are supplied respectively by the posterior branch of the obturator and tibial portion of the sciatic nerves). There are anterior and posterior, but no medial and lateral branches of the obturator nerve. The nerve to obturator internus briefly exits the pelvis via the greater sciatic foramen, giving off a branch to gemellus superior before re-entering the pelvis via the lesser sciatic foramen; it is therefore not at risk during the medial approach to the hip.

18. **B** Convention divides the muscles of the sole of the foot into four layers:

1st Layer	– Abductor hallucis
	– Flexor digitorum brevis
	– Abductor digiti minimi
2nd Layer	– Quadratus plantae
	– Lumbricals
	– Flexor hallucis longus tendon
	– Flexor digitorum longus tendon

3rd Layer	– Flexor hallucis brevis
	– Flexor digiti minimi
	– Adductor hallucis
4th Layer	– Interossei
	– Peroneus longus tendon
	– Tibialis posterior tendon

19. C The long head of the biceps in conjunction with the rotator cuff provides a dynamic component to the stability of the glenohumeral joint. The various ligaments provide different static restraints according to the position of the shoulder:

Ligament	Shoulder position	Movement resisted
Coracohumeral and superior glenohumeral ligaments	Flexion/Int. rotation/abduction Adduction	Posterior translation External rotation/inferior translation
Middle glenohumeral ligament	Adduction/External rotation Mid-abduction (45°)	External rotation Antero-posterior translation
Inferior glenohumeral ligament	45°-90° abduction	Inferior and antero-posterior translation Primary restraint to anterior dislocation – limits ER in abduction (anterior portion) Limits posterior translation in abduction and IR (posterior portion)

20. E The sustentaculum tali is an eminence situated on the anteromedial aspect of the os calcis. Its superior surface forms a support for the middle of the three calcaneal articular facets, all of which articulate with the talus. The flexor hallucis longus tendon passes along a groove on the inferior surface of the sustentaculum. The sustentaculum gives rise to the plantar calcaneo-navicular (spring) ligament, tibiocalcaneal ligament and medial talocalcaneal ligament. The tibial nerve and posterior tibial artery pass through the tarsal tunnel behind the medial malleolus, but their anatomy is unrelated to that of the sustentaculum.

21. D The common peroneal nerve is one of the terminal branches of the sciatic nerve, from which it arises approximately two-thirds of the way down the thigh. Its commonest course is to traverse the popliteal fossa along the medial border of biceps femoris and the fibular attachment of soleus before winding around the fibular neck before dividing into the deep and superficial peroneal nerves within the substance of peroneus longus.

The small saphenous vein is medial to the sural nerve. The popliteal artery lies deep to the popliteal vein which is itself deep to the tibial nerve. Five genicular arteries arise from the popliteal artery – medial and lateral superior genicular arteries, medial and lateral inferior genicular arteries, but only a single middle genicular artery. The popliteal artery initially lies medial to the popliteal vein, but crosses to lie lateral to it as it continues into the calf.

22. C The suboccipital triangle is bounded medially by rectus capitis posterior major and minor, laterally by obliquus capitis superior and inferiorly by obliquus capitis inferior. The great occipital nerve (posterior primary ramus of C2) travels from inferior to superior directly across the superficial aspect of the triangle. The vertebral artery lies in the floor of the triangle on the superior border of the atlas; it is particularly at risk during dissection of the posterior atlantoaxial membrane, through which it enters the spinal canal.

23. B Flexor digitorum profundus arises from the medial aspect of the olecranon process, the proximal 70% of the anterior and medial aspects of the ulnar shaft and part of the adjacent interosseous membrane. The four tendons arise above the wrist (that to the index finger more proximally than the remainder) and pass deep to the flexor digitorum superficialis tendons as all eight together enter the hand deep to the flexor retinaculum. The superficialis tendons each divide into medial and lateral slips through which the respective profundus tendon passes before inserting into the base of the distal phalanx. The medial half of the muscle is innervated by the ulnar nerve, the lateral half by the anterior interosseous branch of the median nerve. There is a secondary role in flexing the wrist but not in supination of the forearm.

24. C The posterolateral approach to the ankle utilises a plane between peroneus brevis (superficial peroneal nerve) and flexor hallucis longus (tibial nerve); the latter is identifiable medially as the most lateral of the deep calf flexor group, and the only one that is still muscular at the level of the distal tibia ("beef to the heel").

Neither peroneus tertius nor tibialis posterior is encountered during this approach. Peroneus longus is identifiable by the fact that it runs posteriorly to peroneus brevis as both pass behind the lateral malleolus; brevis is muscular at this level whilst longus has become tendinous.

25. C The anatomical orientation of the distal humerus is central to the function of the elbow joint; the valgus angulation of the distal humerus contributes toward the carrying of the elbow (5–10° in males, 10-15° in females), whilst the anterior angulation is a factor in the 150° range of flexion. 60% of the axial load is transmitted through the radiocapitellar joint. Proximally, the humeral head is retroverted by 30° relative to the transepicondylar axis.

26. C Each of the lateral aspects of the bodies of the lower cervical vertebrae gives rise to a superior projection known as the uncinate process. These articulate with the neighbouring disc and adjacent vertebral body to form the uncovertebral joints of Luschka from C3 to C7 (although these are claimed by some authors only to occur as a pathological entity in the presence of cervical spondylosis). Neither of the longitudinal ligaments is in any way connected to the uncinate process. The uncinate processes are important landmarks during surgery, as the vertebral arteries lie immediately laterally.

27. A The dorsal columns of the spinal cord transmit ipsilateral sensation to vibration, light touch and proprioception, whilst that to pain and temperature ascends in the contralateral spinothalamic tract. The anterior corticospinal tracts transmit ipsilateral motor impulses before crossing in the anterior white commisure. Conversely the lateral corticospinal tracts decussate in the medulla. A knowledge of these tracts is essential to understanding the features of the different incomplete cord injuries.

28. D The two incision fasciotomy technique involves decompression of lateral and anterior compartments through a single incision 2 cm anterior to the fibular shaft; a second incision 2 cm posterior to the palpable posteromedial edge of the tibia allows decompression of the superficial and deep posterior compartments. There is no medial fascial compartment in the lower leg.

29. E The lateral cutaneous nerve of forearm is the terminal sensory branch of the musculocutaneous nerve. It emerges between biceps and brachialis to cross the cubital fossa superficially before travelling superficially along the radial side of the forearm terminating in the skin overlying the radial artery and anatomical snuff box at the level of the radial styloid. The median nerve and brachial artery are both medial to the biceps tendon, whilst the radial nerve remains deeps first to brachialis then to brachioradialis as it traverses the fossa lateral to biceps. The basilic vein, like all veins, has tributaries but not branches.

30. A The boundaries of the femoral triangle are the inguinal ligament superiorly, the medial border of adductor longus medially and the medial border of sartorius laterally. From lateral to medial the floor comprises iliacus, psoas major, pectineus and adductor longus, and the triangle contains the femoral neurovascular bundle along with the deep inguinal lymph nodes.

31. D The conjoined tendon comprises the combined origins of coracobrachialis and the short head of biceps from the coracoid process of the scapula. Both these muscles take their nerve supply from the musculocutaneous nerve, which arises from the lateral cord of the brachial plexus to enter coracobrachialis from its medial side and actually pass through its substance. Lateral retraction of the tendon therefore carries a high risk of musculocutaneous nerve injury and should be avoided, even if the coracoid is osteotomised.

The upper and lower subscapular nerves arise from the posterior cord so are away from the operative field, as are the lateral pectoral nerve and the lateral thoracic artery; the latter arising from the second part of the axillary artery behind pectoralis minor.

Placement of instrumentation or retractors medial to the conjoined tendon also risks injury to the brachial plexus.

32. A Degenerative spondylolisthesis is commonest at the L4/L5 level, although may occur elsewhere in the lumbosacral spine. Radiculopathy of the L5 nerve root is common due to compression in the lateral recess between the inferior articular facet of L4 and the superior body of L5. This may lead to reduced power in extensors hallucis and digitorum longus, as well as altered sensation on the dorsum of the foot. EHL and the first web space are exclusively inner-vated by L5. In most cases neither Achilles (S1) nor patellar (L4) tendon reflexes are noticeably affected.

33. **A** The extensor musculature of the back is essential to the main-tenance of normal posture and is arranged in three layers. The deepest layer comprises short muscles – interspinales and intertransversarii – which run between spinous and transverse processes of adjacent vertebrae. An intermediate layer of longer oblique muscles also connects the spinous and transverse processes; this layer comprises the semispinalis, multifidus and rotators which together make up the trans-versospinalis. Most superficially, the erector spinae group runs longitu-dinally along the entire length of the spine – its constituents are iliocostalis, longissimus and spinalis (each subdivided; see for example longissimus thoracis, cervicis and capitis).

34. **D** The normal facial appearance excludes a pre-ganglionic injury, which would result in features of a Horner's syndrome. The classic 'waiter's tip' deformity is diagnostic of an upper plexus injury affecting C5 and C6 +/- C7 (Erb-Duchenne). A lower plexus injury (Klumpke's) is characterised by clawing of the hand, which results from paralysis of the intrinsic muscles. Combined upper and lower plexus injury is usually associated with significant trauma; all sensory and motor function in the affected limb is lost. Isolated avulsion of the suprascapular nerve (which supplies supraspinatus and infraspinatus) is not known.

35. **B** Other than its role in limiting abduction of the metacarpals, the chief relevance of the natatory ligament is its involvement in the pathoanatomy of Dupuytren's contracture. Also known as the superfi-cial transverse metacarpal ligament, the natatory ligament runs between the metacarpophalangeal joints, lying immediately beneath the volar skin of the web spaces. All structures passing from the hand into the finger therefore lie deep (dorsal) to the ligament.

Extended Matching Answers

1. I The suprascapular nerve arises from the upper trunk and travels laterally under omohyoid and trapezius to pass under the superior transverse scapular ligament into the supraspinous fossa where it supplies supraspinatus. It finally curves around the lateral border of the scapular spine to give off small branches to the glenohumeral joint capsule, before terminating in the infraspinous fossa where it supplies infraspinatus.

2. A In addition to pectoralis minor, coracobrachialis and the short head of biceps, several ligaments attach to the coracoid process – coracoacromial, coracohumeral and the two coracoclavicular ligaments; conoid and trapezoid. The trapezoid is the more lateral of the two. The acromioclavicular joint is also stabilised distally by its own joint capsule and the acromioclavicular ligament.

3. D In addition to the static stabilisation afforded by the joint congruity, labrum, coracohumeral and three glenohumeral ligaments, the shoulder joint receives dynamic stabilisation from the rotator cuff muscles and the long head of biceps. The latter also has a weak role in depressing the humeral head.

4. F Rhomboid major originates from the spines of the T2–T5 vertebrae and the overlying supraspinous ligaments. Its insertion is into the medial border of the scapula medial to the infraspinous fossa (almost entirely filled by infraspinatus). Immediately anterior to this point of attachment, serratus anterior also inserts along the medial border of the scapula. Levator scapulae also inserts into the medial border of the scapula, but more superiorly.

5. J The upper subscapular nerve arises immediately the posterior cord is formed from the three posterior divisions. It is the sole nerve supply to subscapularis. The lower branch also innervates teres major.

6. C The radial nerve divides anterior to the lateral epicondyle to give its terminal superficial radial and posterior interosseous branches. The posterior interosseous nerve passes between (and supplies) the deep and superficial heads of supinator to enter the posterior compartment, where it innervates all the extensors except for extensor carpi radialis longus (supplied by the radial nerve).

7. **D** The median nerve passes medial to the brachial artery in the anticubital fossa, giving off an articular branch prior to exiting the fossa and entering the forearm via the two heads of pronator teres. Consequently pronator syndrome gives motor and sensory median nerve symptoms.

8. **D** See answer 9.

9. **H** The median nerve exits the cubital fossa between the humeral and ulnar heads of pronator teres; the ulnar head separates it from the ulnar artery. At the inferior border of the humeral head the median nerve gives off an important branch, the anterior interosseous nerve, to supply flexor pollicis longus, the lateral half of flexor digitorum profundus, pronator quadratus and part of the wrist capsule. The median nerve itself continues distally on the belly of flexor digitorum profundus, and covered by flexor digitorum superficialis, before passing into the palm of the hand within the flexor retinaculum; it provides sensory innervation to lateral aspect of the hand, as well as motor function to the 'LOAF' muscles (1st and 2nd lumbricals, opponens pollicis, abductor pollicis brevis and flexor pollicis brevis).

10. **G** Four muscles form the superficial group taking origin from the medial epicondyle. From medial to lateral these are: flexor carpi ulnaris, palmaris longus, flexor carpi radialis and pronator teres. Deep to this, the flexor digitorum superficialis also takes origin from the medial epicondyle.

Chapter 2
Imaging Techniques

MCQ 20
EMQ 5

Multiple Choice Questions

1. All of the following structures appear dark on both T1- and T2-weighted MRI EXCEPT:
   a. Cortical bone
   b. Fibrocartilage
   c. Hyaline cartilage
   d. Tendon
   e. Ligament

2. Which of the following statements regarding ultrasound scanning is TRUE?
   a. Fluid-filled cavities are very echogenic on ultrasound
   b. Ultrasound waves are generated by passing electromagnetic waves through piezoelectric crystals
   c. Ultrasound operates in the frequency range 80–350 MHz
   d. Higher frequencies give greater wave attenuation as ultrasound passes through tissues
   e. Lower frequency ultrasound waves give greater image resolution

3. **How is the Z-score for bone mineral density (BMD) calculated following Dual Energy X-ray Absorptiometry (DEXA) scanning?**
    a. $$\frac{\text{Patient's BMD} - \text{Peak BMD for young adult of same sex}}{\text{Standard deviation of peak BMD for population}}$$
    b. $$\frac{\text{Patient's BMD} - \text{BMD for adult of same sex and age}}{\text{Standard deviation of age-adjusted BMD for population}}$$
    c. $$\frac{\text{Peak BMD for young adult of same sex} - \text{Patient's BMD}}{\text{Standard deviation of peak BMD for population}}$$
    d. $$\frac{\text{BMD for adult of same sex and age} - \text{Patient's BMD}}{\text{Standard deviation of age-adjusted BMD for population}}$$
    e. $$\frac{\text{Patient's BMD} - \text{Standard deviation of peak BMD for population}}{\text{Peak BMD for young adult of same sex}}$$

4. **What is the World Health Organisation definition of osteoporosis?**
    a. T-score between -1 and -2.5
    b. T-score less than -2.5
    c. T-score less than -2.5 plus at least one fragility fracture
    d. Z-score between -1 and -2.5
    e. Z-score less than -2.5

5. **Which of the following best describes the common mechanism by which x-rays are converted to a digital image by a flat panel detector (FPD)?**
    a. An outer caesium layer on the FPD converts the x-rays to light; a silicon photodiode then converts this light to an electric current which generates a screen image
    b. The FPD contains a tungsten filament which generates a current as it is struck by x-rays; this current is then converted to an image by the computer software
    c. The FPD contains a caesium photodiode which generates an electric current when struck by x-radiation; software then converts this current to a screen image
    d. An outer silver iodobromide layer on the FPD converts the x-rays to light; a tungsten photodiode then converts this light to an electric current which generates a screen image
    e. An outer piezoelectric layer on the FPD converts the x-rays to micro-sound waves; a further inner piezoelectric layer then converts this to an electric current which generates a screen image

6. **Which of the following pathological conditions appears cold on ^{99}technetium bone-scanning?**
   a. Paget's disease
   b. Multiple myeloma
   c. Osteoarthritis
   d. Osteomyelitis
   e. Cervical spondylosis

7. **Which of the following statements regarding proton precession in the context of MRI scanning is TRUE?**
   a. Precession refers to the frequency at which protons rotate around their longitudinal axis
   b. T1 weighting is defined by the time taken for precession to regain 63% of its maximum value
   c. T2 weighting is defined by the time taken for precession to fall to 37% of its maximum value
   d. The application of a radiofrequency pulse to the patient causes the precessions of all protons within the field to fall into phase
   e. The application of a magnetic field to the patient causes the precessions of all protons to fall into phase

8. **Which of the following statements regarding ^{67}gallium bone scanning is FALSE?**
   a. ^{67}Ga requires delayed imaging (24–48 hours)
   b. ^{67}Ga scanning is more dependent on blood flow than ^{99}Tc scanning
   c. ^{67}Ga scanning has a role in assessment of sarcoidosis
   d. A *double tracer* technique is frequently employed utilising simultaneous administration of ^{99}Tc and ^{67}Ga
   e. ^{67}Ga Scanning is poor at differentiating between cellulitis and osteomyelitis

9. **What is the approximate CT attenuation coefficient of cortical bone?**
   a. -1000 Hounsfield units
   b. -100 Hounsfield units
   c. 0 Hounsfield units
   d. 100 Hounsfield units
   e. 1000 Hounsfield units

10. **Which is the approximate radiation dose sustained during a single plain radiograph?**
    a. 0.005mSv
    b. 0.05mSv
    c. 0.5mSv
    d. 5mSv
    e. 50mSv

11. **Which of the following is conventionally used to provide contrast in CT scanning?**
    a. Technetium
    b. Iodine
    c. Indium
    d. Gallium
    e. Gadolinium

12. **Which of the following characteristically leads to a falsely high bone mineral density (BMD) score being calculated following DEXA scanning?**
    a. Previous surgical resection of spinal posterior elements
    b. Primary hyperparathyroidism
    c. Osteomalacia
    d. Vertebral osteoarthritis
    e. Aicardi syndrome

13. **Which of the following statements regarding positron emission tomography (PET) is FALSE?**
    a. A positron is a positively charged electron
    b. The short $t_{1/2}$ of the radionuclides used in PET normally necessitates their being produced on site
    c. The image generated results from photon emission when the positron combines with an electron to undergo annihilation
    d. The radionuclide doses required for image detection in PET are considerably higher than those used in other nuclear imaging modalities
    e. The positrons are normally administered to the patient as ^{18}F-fludeoxyglucose

14. **What does *B-mode* stand for in the context of ultrasound scanning?**
    a. Bone mode
    b. Biphasic mode
    c. Brightness mode
    d. Bremsstrahlung mode
    e. Brownian mode

15. **Which of the following best describes the underlying principles of magnetic resonance imaging?**
    a. Rapid electromagnetic pulses are applied to the patient, causing electrons to change both alignment and precession phase; as they do so they generate currents in the receiver coil
    b. Rapid electromagnetic pulses are applied to the patient, causing protons to change alignment; as they do so they generate currents in the receiver coil
    c. Rapid electromagnetic pulses are applied to the patient, causing protons to change precession phase; as they do so they generate currents in the receiver coil
    d. A constant electromagnetic field is applied to the patient; onto this are superimposed radiofrequency pulses, causing protons to change both alignment and precession phase
    e. A constant electromagnetic field is applied to the patient; onto this are superimposed radiofrequency pulses, causing electrons to change both alignment and precession phase

16. **Which of the following findings on technetium bone scanning is most consistent with a diagnosis of avascular necrosis of the femoral head?**
    a. A posteromedial photopaenic region surrounded by a zone of increased activity
    b. A posteromedial zone of increased activity surrounded by a photopaenic region
    c. A central photopaenic zone surrounded by normal bone
    d. An anterosuperior photopaenic region surrounded by a zone of increased activity
    e. An anterosuperior zone of increased activity surrounded by a photopaenic region

17. **Which of the following best describes the mechanism by which x-rays are generated?**
    a. Electrons from a superheated tungsten cathode strike an anode – x-rays are released as this impact takes place
    b. Protons from a superheated tungsten anode strike a cathode – x-rays are released as this impact takes place
    c. Electrons from a superheated tungsten anode strike a cathode – x-rays are released as this impact takes place
    d. A superheated tungsten cathode and anode respectively release electrons and protons – these collide at half the speed of light to release x-rays
    e. A superheated tungsten anode and cathode respectively release electrons and protons – these collide at half the speed of light to release x-rays

18. **Which of the following causes an object (or material) to appear LIGHTER, as opposed to darker, on CT scanning?**
    a. High atomic number
    b. Low atomic number
    c. Increased number of voxels
    d. Positive charge
    e. High water content

19. **Which of the following statements regarding the use of ^{99}technetium in radionuclide bone scanning is FALSE?**
    a. In order to be administered intravenously ^{99}Tc is coupled to a phosphate compound
    b. Nearly three quarters of the administered dose is excreted within the first 24 hours
    c. Decay of ^{99}Tc generates pure γ-radiation
    d. The half-life of ^{99}Tc *in vivo* is approximately 12 hours
    e. ^{99}Tc arises as a result of the decay of the unstable ^{99}Mo isotope.

20. **Which one of the following statements regarding the genera-tion of x-rays within an x-ray machine is TRUE?**

   a. X-radiation is generated by electrons striking a tungsten anode at a speed of 80,000 km s^{-1}
   b. X-radiation is generated by electrons striking a tungsten anode at a speed of 40,000 km s^{-1}
   c. 80% of x-radiation arises from electrons striking nuclei within the anode
   d. 80% of x-radiation arises from electrons striking inner electrons within the anode
   e. 80% of x-radiation arises from electrons striking outer electrons within the anode

Extended Matching Questions

SCENARIO I OPTIONS

A Plain radiograph

B Ultrasound scan

C Duplex untrasound scan

D MARS (metal artefact reduction sequencing) MRI

E Plain MRI

F Radionuclide bone scanning

G Computerised tomography (CT)

H DEXA scanning

I Spiral CT

For each of the following clinical examples, select the most appropriate NEXT radiological investigation from the list above. Each option may be used once, more than once, or not at all.

1. A 2-month-old boy is found to have abnormal findings on undertaking the Ortolani and Barlow tests.

2. A 77-year-old man becomes hypoxic 72 hours following a total knee replacement. His ECG is normal other than showing a mild sinus tachycardia.

3. 3 years following hip resurfacing arthroplasty, a 42-year-old man attends the clinic complaining of groin pain. His inflammatory markers are normal but his serum cobalt is mildly elevated. Plain radiograph is unremarkable.

4. 11 years following total knee replacement, a 74-year-old man attends the clinic complaining of pain in the joint. His inflammatory markers are normal, and plain radiograph is unremarkable.

5. A 57-year-old man is on the waiting list for revision of the acetabular component of a metal-on-polyethylene total hip replacement, implanted 17 years ago. Plain radiographs suggest significant osteolysis around the component, which has migrated superiorly.

Answers: Chapter 2

> MCQ 20
> EMQ 5

Multiple Choice Answers

1. **C** The MRI characteristics of some of the commoner tissues and structures are as follows:

Tissue	T1	T2
Cortical bone	Dark	Dark
Red bone marrow	Grey	Grey
Yellow bone marrow	Bright	Grey
Muscle	Grey	Grey
Tendon	Dark	Dark
Ligament	Dark	Dark
Fibrocartilage	Dark	Dark
Hyaline cartilage	Grey	Grey
Fat	Bright	Grey
Water	Dark	Bright

2. **D** Ultrasound operates in the frequency 3–50MHz, and results from the generation of waves by the passing of an alternating current through a piezoelectric crystal; the waves are then reflected back off different tissues with different intensities. As the crystal is struck by the returning waves a voltage is set up which is converted to an image. Fluid-filled cavities have very low echogenicity, whereas that of fat is high. Higher frequencies give greater image resolution but also greater attenuation as ultrasound waves pass through tissues.

3. **B** The T-score is calculated as:

$$\frac{\text{Patient's BMD} - \text{Peak BMD for young adult of same sex}}{\text{Standard deviation of peak BMD for population}}$$

The Z-score is given by:

$$\frac{\text{Patient's BMD} - \text{BMD for adult of same sex and age}}{\text{Standard deviation of age-adjusted BMD for population}}$$

A low Z-score (i.e. BMD is low even against the age-matched population) is suggestive of underlying pathology other than simple age-related osteoporosis.

4. B The WHO criterion for the definition of osteoporosis is based on a T-score of less than -2.5. If one or more fragility fractures are present in addition, *severe* osteoporosis is diagnosed. A T-score between -1 and -2.5 gives a diagnosis of osteopaenia. Z-scores are not part of these definitions.

5. A Most digital x-ray imaging is obtained via the use of a flat panel detector (FPD). Most FPDs have an outer caesium layer and a deeper silicon photodiode layer. As the x-radiation strikes the caesium, light is generated; the photodiode then converts this to a current, which in turn generates an image. Although this is easy and convenient as compared with 'old style' x-ray films, some resolution is lost in the process.

6. B ^{99}Tc bone scanning is effectively a measure of osteoblast activity; images are timed at three different phases – dynamic (1–2 minutes), blood pool (30 minutes) and static (4 hours). The conditions that classically appear cold are bone islands (enostoses), multiple myeloma, and skeletal metastases from renal and thyroid malignancies. Osteomyelitis is characterised by the fact that it appears hot on all three phases.

7. D Precession refers to the wobble of a proton (or other particle) around its longitudinal axis. MRI scanning starts with the application of a magnetic field to the patient; this causes all protons to align along the longitudinal axis of the scanner. Radiofrequency pulses are then super-imposed on the magnetic field; these have a dual effect, the first of which is to alter the alignment of the protons such that they are now at a transverse angle to the longitudinal axis, and the second is to bring the precessions of all protons into phase with one another. When the pulse is discontinued, these processes reverse. T1 weighting is defined by the time taken for the longitudinal magnetisation vector to regain 63% of its maximum value, whilst T2 refers to the time delay for the transverse magnetisation vector to fall to 37% of its maximum value.

8. B ^{67}Ga is a radionuclide that may be used in bone scanning as an alternative to ^{99}Tc; indeed, the two are often used together as a *double tracer* technique. One of its strengths lies in the fact that it is less dependent on blood flow than ^{99}Tc scanning, and thus may identify foci not seen with ^{99}Tc; this also forms part of the explanation for its value in the assessment of granulomatous diseases such as tuberculosis and sarcoidosis. It is poor at differentiating cellulitis from osteomyelitis, however, and requires delayed imaging at 24–48 hours, potentially even up to a week.

9. E Computerised tomography (CT) is based on similar principles to standard x-ray, but the use of a rotating x-ray tube and accurate receptors gives a far greater degree of resolution and allows cross-sectional 'cuts' to be obtained. Different tissue types have different *attenuation coefficients* which result in some appearing much denser than others on CT (a higher attenuation coefficient leads to a denser appearance).

Tissue	Attenuation coefficient (Hounsfield units)
Air	–1000
Fat	–100
Water	0
Soft tissue	50–100
Bone	1000

10. B The sievert (Sv) is the SI derived unit of dose equivalent radiation; unlike the gray (Gy) it aims to take account of the biological effect of the radiation rather than merely the actual dose. However, for x-rays and gamma rays, the two are equivalent. A plain radiograph provides a dose of approximately 0.05mSv, as opposed to 3.5mSv with a spinal CT and 5.0 mSv in patients undergoing radionuclide bone scanning.

11. B The contrast media used in CT scanning and plain x-ray are iodine based, as opposed to those in MRI, which most commonly use gadolinium. ^{99}Technetium, ^{111}indium and ^{67}gallium are all used in radionuclide bone scanning.

12. **D** Osteoarthritis can lead to a falsely high BMD calculation due to associated sclerotic changes. BMD over-estimation may also result following vertebral body fractures. Hyperparathyroidism causes a reduction in bone mass, whilst posterior element resection leads to an under-estimation of BMD. Osteomalacia is characterised by impaired mineralisation of bone, and may reduce BMD, but does not give a false estimate. Aicardi syndrome affects the central nervous system with no known involvement of the skeleton.

13. **D** PET scanning uses radio-isotopes which undergo decay to produce positrons (positively charged electrons). These are usually administered as the glucose analogue 18F-fludeoxyglucose, and so become concentrated at areas of high metabolic activity – including sites of malignancy.

Each positron undergoes annihilation when it combines with a free electron, a process which releases photons; these form the basis of the image generation. The short half-life of the radionuclides usually requires on-site production. PET is particularly sensitive, and so requires lower doses than other forms of nuclear imaging.

14. **C** The three main modes in which ultrasound scanning may be used are A-mode (amplitude mode), B-mode (brightness mode) and M-mode (time-motion mode). B-mode is the most widely undertaken, and can be used to produce images such as those familiar to the orthopaedic surgeon in the assessment of developmental dysplasia of the hip.

15. **D** In the MRI scanner a steady magnetic field is applied to the patient, which causes the protons both to align themselves along the field, and to fall into precession phase (precession refers to the wobble of a proton around its longitudinal axis). Bursts of radiofrequency are then applied to the patient, which cause both the precession phase and alignment to alter. As the radiofrequency burst finishes, the phase and alignment revert, thereby inducing a current in the receiving coil – which in turn leads to the generation of an image.

16. **D** Although to an extent MRI is superseding radionuclide bone scanning in the assessment of femoral head AVN, the latter is still a valuable diagnostic tool. The static images show increased uptake in the layer of reactive bone at the periphery of the infarction zone, which is itself visible as a photopaenic (cold) area in the area of avascular necrosis. Classically this is seen within the hip in the anterosuperior region of the femoral head.

17. A See question 20 for explanation.

18. A High atomic (or molecular) number causes tissues to have a higher attenuation coefficient, and therefore appear lighter, on CT scanning. Charge does not affect this. Water has a lower attenuation coefficient than solid material and therefore does not increase the brightness of a material on CT. The voxel is the three-dimensional equivalent of the pixel and is not a property of matter.

19. D ^{99}Tc is generated by decay of the ^{99}Mo isotope. For injection, it is usually coupled with methylene diphosphonate; this causes it to be incorporated into hydroxyapatite in bone, and thus to become concentrated around areas of increased osteoblastic activity. A γ-camera is used to generate an image. Excretion is renal; approximately 70–75% is excreted within the first 24 hours. The $t_{1/2}$ of ^{99}Tc is roughly 6 hours.

20. C The first stage in the generation of x-radiation within an x-ray machine is the release of free electrons into a vacuum from a tungsten cathode heated to 2200°C. These are drawn towards a positively charged tungsten anode at approximately 140,000 km s^{-1} – as they strike the tungsten, both heat and x-radiation are generated. 80% of this x-radiation arises from electrons striking the tungsten nuclei; the remaining 20% from electrons striking inner electrons which are then pushed into outer orbital levels.

Extending Matching Answers

1. **B**
2. **I**
3. **D**
4. **F**
5. **G**

The Ortolani and Barlow tests between them are virtually diagnostic of developmental dysplasia of the hip; the investigation of choice for this is ultrasound scanning, which effectively assesses the degree of coverage of the head.

Following any form of lower limb surgery, sudden hypoxia should alert a high index of suspicion of pulmonary embolism; spiral CT of the chest has now largely superseded ventilation-perfusion scanning as the investigation of choice in such circumstances.

The MHRA has set out fairly clear guidelines for the management of the painful metal-on-metal hip prosthesis; in addition to plain films and blood test, MARS MRI should be considered in all such patients to investigate the possibility of fluid accumulation and exclude the possibility of a pseudotumour (Pandit *et al*, *JBJS-B* 2008).

In the investigation of other painful prostheses, however, the imaging of choice after plain radiography remains radionuclide bone scanning, which will assess for both infection and aseptic loosening.

Where a significant bony defect is suspected prior to revision hip arthroplasty, especially on the acetabular side, CT scans obtained before the day of surgery provide invaluable information about the extent of any acetabular defects, and allow accurate preoperative planning to be undertaken.

Chapter 3

Bone, Bone Grafting and Fracture Healing

MCQ 15
EMQ 14

Multiple Choice Questions

1. What % of the dry weight of bone is composed of inorganic material?
   a. 10%
   b. 20%
   c. 40%
   d. 70%
   e. 90%

2. Which one of the following mechanisms will lead to a fracture with the lowest applied force?
   a. Shear
   b. Tension
   c. Compression
   d. Strain
   e. Bending

3. What kind of fracture healing occurs in a minimally displaced oblique fibula fracture treated non-operatively?
   a. Primary fracture healing
   b. Secondary fracture healing
   c. Direct healing
   d. Intramembranous ossification
   e. Remodelling healing

4. **Which one of the following statements about woven bone is FALSE?**
   a. Woven bone is found in the foetus
   b. Woven bone can be found in the adult
   c. Woven bone contains up to eight times as many osteocytes as the same volume of lamellar bone
   d. Woven bone has a lower Young's modulus than lamellar bone
   e. Woven bone has Haversian canals

5. **Regarding bone grafts, which one of the following statements is FALSE?**
   a. Vascularisation precedes creeping substitution
   b. Allograft incorporates more slowly than autograft
   c. Washing allograft decreases its rate of incorporation
   d. Washing autograft makes no difference to its rate of incorporation
   e. HIV can be transmitted by allograft

6. **Which one of the following mechanical properties of bone graft is not affected by irradiation?**
   a. Young's modulus
   b. Bone strength
   c. Work to fracture
   d. Resistance to crack propagation
   e. Fatigue life

7. **Which of the following bone graft materials is normally still visible on plain radiographs five years after implantation?**
   a. Cancellous autograft
   b. Cancellous allograft
   c. Beta tricalcium phosphate
   d. Hydroxyapatite
   e. Demineralised bone matrix (DBX)

8. **Regarding cells found in bone, which one of the following is FALSE?**

   a. Osteocytes are the commonest cell found within adult bone
   b. Osteoblasts express RANKL
   c. Bisphosphonates act on osteoclasts
   d. Osteoblasts have a ruffled border
   e. Osteoblasts are the only bone cell to have a receptor for PTH

9. **Which of the following is the most accurate response about the mechanical properties of adult human lamellar bone?**

   a. It is isotropic
   b. Fatigue failure is not affected by temperature
   c. Cancellous bone is stronger in tension than in compression
   d. It demonstrates hysteresis
   e. It becomes stiffer at lower rates of strain

10. **In secondary (biologic) fracture healing, which one of the following responses is INCORRECT?**

    a. Type II collagen is laid down before type I collagen
    b. Oxygen tension is high in newly formed callus
    c. The highest oxygen tension occurs in granulation tissue
    d. Type I collagen is laid down in the remodelling phase
    e. As the fracture heals the strain across the fracture fragments decreases

11. **Regarding intramedullary nailing of long bone fractures, which of the following is the most accurate statement?**

    a. The blood supply after reaming returns to normal in one month
    b. The blood supply after reaming is centripetal
    c. Reaming decreases the blood supply by less than 50%
    d. An intramedullary nail acts as a load bearing device
    e. Nails that fit more tightly against the cortex do not interfere more with revascularisation

12. **Which one of the following statements about allograft is TRUE?**
    a. Freezing makes little difference to the mechanical properties
    b. Freeze drying makes little difference to the mechanical properties
    c. Cortical strut allograft incorporates at the same rate as cancellous graft
    d. Removal of cartilage makes no difference to the biomechanical properties of the graft
    e. Allograft has osteogenic properties

13. **Which one of the following is the most important factor in increasing stability in external fixators?**
    a. Number of pins used
    b. Proximity of pins to fracture site
    c. The bone–frame distance
    d Number of bars used
    e. Diameter of the pins

14. **Which one of the following substances is used primarily for its osteoinductive role?**
    a. Allograft
    b. Demineralised bone matrix
    c. Autograft
    d. Hydroxyapatite
    e. Beta tricalcium phosphate

15. **Which one of the following statements is NOT true about the blood supply to bone?**
    a. Bone receives up to 20% of cardiac output
    b. Blood supply only crosses a growth plate in a child
    c. The physis has a slow blood flow
    d. Intravascular pressure is greater in the medullary canal than in the periosteum
    e. The venous drainage of bone is almost solely to the periosteum

Extended Matching Questions

SCENARIO I OPTIONS

A Increases two times

B Increases four times

C Increases eight times

D Halves

E No effect

F Decreases four times

G Increases sixteen times

Which answer best fits the questions below? Each option may be used once, more than once or not at all.

1. What is the effect on bending stiffness of doubling the thickness of a steel plate?

2. If the thickness of a titanium and a steel plate are both doubled, by how much does the bending stiffness of the steel plate increase compared to the titanium plate?

3. If the width of a plate is doubled, what is the effect upon bending stiffness?

4. If the working length of a plate is doubled, what is the effect upon bending stiffness?

5. If the working length of a nail is doubled, what is the effect upon bending stiffness?

6. If the working length of a nail is doubled, what is the effect upon torsional stiffness?

7. If the diameter of a solid nail is doubled, what is the effect upon bending stiffness?

8. If the diameter of a solid nail is doubled, what is the effect upon torsional stiffness?

SCENARIO II OPTIONS

A	200%	**F**	10%
B	100%	**G**	2%
C	50%	**H**	1%
D	30%	**I**	0%
E	20%		

The following questions refer to fracture healing. For each of the questions, select the most correct option. Each option may be used once, more than once or not at all. However, for each question there is only one correct answer from the list of options.

9. What is the maximum strain at a fracture to allow the formation of granulation tissue?

10. What is the maximum strain at a fracture to allow the formation of woven bone?

11. What is the maximum strain at a fracture to allow the formation of lamellar bone?

12. A patient is seen in fracture clinic 6 months following intramedullary nailing of his femur. Radiographs demonstrate resorption at the fracture site, and no evidence of bone healing. He has normal biology and is otherwise well with no evidence of infection. What is the strain at the fracture site?

13. The same patient undergoes exchange nailing from an 8 mm to 12 mm nail following which the painful clicking disappears. He is seen in fracture clinic 12 weeks after revision and some callus is seen on the radiographs – what is the strain now?

14. He attends for final follow up 2 years later and has remodelled his femur. What is the maximum strain the fracture site can withstand?

Answers: Chapter 3

MCQ 15
EMQ 14

Multiple Choice Answers

1. D   The inorganic or mineral phase of bone makes up 70% of the dry weight. The mineral phase is composed mainly of calcium phosphate, often in the form of hydroxyapatite and a smaller proportion of calcium carbonate. The organic component makes up the remaining 30% of the dry weight. It is composed mainly of type I collagen.

2. A   Bone is weakest in shear and strongest in compression due to the alignment of the Haversian canals. A bending force results in the creation of a transverse fracture. The convex side of the bone fails first due to the tension load. The fracture then propagates to the other cortex. With greater applied energy a butterfly fragment becomes more prominent on the compression side and the degree of comminution increases. Strain is defined as change in length over initial length, and is not a mechanism of failure.

3. B   A fracture that is anatomically reduced and fixed with absolute stability (less than 50 μm relative motion) between the bone ends will heal with primary fracture healing. The fracture heals without callus with the cutting cones crossing the fracture gap and 'remodelling' the fracture site without interruption. By contrast, secondary fracture healing occurs when there is relative stability, generating a stimulus to fracture healing and callus formation. This follows the laying down of cartilage and therefore ossifies by endochondral ossification.

4. E   Lamellar (mature) bone is subdivided into cortical and cancellous bone depending on its three dimensional structure. It is not found in the foetus. Haversian systems are the functional units of lamellar bone. By contrast woven (immature) bone is found in the foetus, fracture healing (before remodelling), and in pathological states, e.g. Paget's disease.

Woven bone has a more disorganised structure than lamellar bone, is more cellular (up to eight times that of lamellar bone) and more metabolically active.

5. D Bone grafts are incorporated by a process of creeping substitution. In cancellous bone graft there is firstly revascularisation of the bone. In the case of autograft this happens very quickly, allograft takes longer. Osteoblasts then lay down new osteoid on the dead trabeculae. There is plenty of space in the trabeculae to allow neovascularisation and the laying down of osteoid. This old necrotic bone is then slowly remodelled by osteoclasts. Due to the surface area of the trabeculae this process usually reaches completion faster than with cortical graft.

In the case of cortical grafts there is slower revascularisation which occurs through the old Haversian and Volkmann canals beginning peripherally. Some areas may never obtain a blood supply. The bone has to be reabsorbed to make room for the deposited osteoid; this process is very slow. Neobone is often laid down on the periphery and cortical grafts may become incorporated by new bone rather than remodelled. The process in cortical and structural grafts may be incomplete.

Washing of allograft increases its speed of incorporation whereas the washing of autograft decreases its speed of incorporation. HIV can be transmitted by allograft, even when irradiated up to 25 kGy.

6. A With a standard dose of 25 kGy of gamma irradiation there are significant decreases in bone strength, work to fracture, and impact energy absorption, reduction in fatigue life of the bone and a reduction in the resistance to crack propagation; but no effect upon the Young's modulus.

7. D Cancellous auto- and allograft become incorporated quickly. Cancellous autograft becomes incorporated faster than cancellous allograft but in both remodelling is usually complete. Beta tricalcium phosphate under goes dissolution quickly and this limits use in structural situations. DBX is not visible on radiographs. Remodelling of hydroxyapatite is very slow and is usually incomplete.

8. D   Osteocytes are the commonest cell within adult bone and are derived from osteoblasts that have become trapped within lacunae in bone. They are surrounded by concentric lamellae and communicate with neighbouring osteocytes by canaliculi.

The osteoclast is a multinucleated cell derived from a monocyte lineage and functions to reabsorb/remodel bone. The ruffled border allows attachment of the osteoclast to the surface of bone through the anchorin-integrin mechanism. Bisphosphonates act on osteoclasts through inhibiting the formation of the ruffled border or by causing apoptosis. Calcitonin, not PTH, acts on the osteoclast.

Osteoblasts are responsible for the laying down of bone matrix after the osteoclast has resorbed the bone. They have PTH receptors. After PTH has bound to the receptor the osteoblast expresses Receptor Activator of Nuclear Factor kB Ligand (RANK-L). RANK-L in turn binds to its receptor Receptor Activator of Nuclear Factor kB (RANK) on the osteoclast which leads to its activation.

9. D   Lamellar bone is viscoelastic and demonstrates hysteresis, rate sensitivity (becoming stiffer with increasing rate of strain), it exhibits creep with application of a constant stress and undergoes stress relaxation. In addition its mechanical properties are affected by hydration and temperature. It is stronger in compression than tension and has anisotropic properties.

10. B   The stages of fracture healing are:

Inflammation – a haematoma is produced immediately after the fracture. This serves to provide some of the pluripotent cells for fracture healing and secretes growth factors. Fibroblasts migrate into the fracture site and start to lay down granulation tissue. Granulation tissue can tolerate the greatest strain, at this moment there is the greatest oxygen tension.

Soft Callus Formation – Primary soft callus is formed within 2 weeks of the fracture. Stability of the fracture increases, decreasing the strain across the fracture gap. Type II collagen is at a high concentration 9 days after the fracture. Subsequently type I collagen expression increases. Type X collagen is expressed by hypertrophic chondrocytes during the calcification of the extraarticular matrix.

Hard Callus Formation – Endochondral ossification converts soft callus to hard callus (woven bone). Medullary callus also supplements the bridging soft callus. These processes further decrease the strain at the fracture site. Newly formed callus has low oxygen tension.

Remodelling – starts as soon as the fracture site is bridged and can carry on for many years.

11. B The insertion of any intramedullary device (eg nail) decreases the intramedullary blood supply, particularly in the case of reamed nails. Cortical revascularisation occurs twice as fast following unreamed nailing compared with reamed nailing with no difference detectable at 12 weeks. After reaming the blood supply becomes centripetal rather than centrifugal (known as reversal). There is a much greater increase in the periosteal circulation with reamed nailing.

A nail acts as a load sharing device with the surrounding bone, if the fracture ends are in contact.

12. A Freezing makes no difference to the mechanical properties whereas freeze drying makes the bone more brittle (inducing microfractures). Strut allograft may never incorporate and its use is associated with infection, non-union and fracture. Removal of cartilage from bone graft is a biomechanically and histologically important step, with its inclusion resulting in lower graft stiffness and lack of remodelling seen in areas where the cartilage is present. Allograft has osteoconductive properties only.

13. E All of the answers increase stability of a fixator but the single greatest contributor is fracture reduction. Of the options listed, however, pin diameter has the greatest effect (proportional to radius[4]). Larger diameter pins provide a more rigid fixator, which in turn provides less bending stress at the bone-pin interface. However, the hole size acts as a stress riser; if the pin diameter is greater than 30% the diameter of the bone then the risk of fracture through the hole after pin removal greatly increases.

External fixator stability can be increased by:
- Increasing the pin diameter
- Increasing the number of pins
- Increasing the spread of the pins
- Multiplanar fixation
- Reducing the bone-frame distance
- Multiple bars stacked in height
- Reducing the working distance
- Use of olive wires
- Use of stainless steel rings/bars rather than titanium

14. B Terms that are frequently tested in the exam are:

Osteoconductive – a scaffold upon which bone can grow

Osteoinductive – factors that can induce undifferentiated cells to become active osteoblasts

Osteogenic – living bone cells within the tissue capable of producing bone

Allograft is derived from another individual of the same species. It has osteoconductive properties and acts as a scaffold for host bone. It has no osteoinductive or osteogenic properties. Xenograft is graft derived from another species. Autograft is derived from the same individual.

Demineralised bone matrix is allograft treated with acid to remove the inorganic material to leave the organic materials and growth factors. It provides better osteoinductivity than undemineralised allograft. However, it has no structural properties.

Autograft is derived from the same individual – it is osteogenic, osteoinductive and osteoconductive. It is the gold standard against which all other graft materials are compared.

Hydroxyapatite and beta tricalcium phosphate are bioceramics that have osteoconductive properties but no osteoinductive or osteogenic properties. They are useful for filling bone defects.

15. B Up to 20% of cardiac output is used to supply bone. Blood supply never crosses the physis which accounts for the need for separate blood supplies to epiphysis and diaphysis. The physis is supplied from the periosteal blood supply at the metaphysis, which penetrates the bone and links with the diaphyseal blood supply. This network supplies the physis via vessels that have a hairpin bend adjacent to the physis which serves to slow the blood flow. The growth plate in the child is not crossed by vessels. Intravascular pressure is greater in the medullary canal than in the periosteum and therefore the inner two-thirds is supplied by the medullary supply and the outer one-third is supplied by the periosteal supply. The venous system of bone virtually all drains towards the periosteum.

Extending Matching Answers

1. C

2. E

3. A

4. F

The effect of the load on a beam in terms of its deflection is a popular question. If a force is applied to the end of a plate, then the predominant deflection is bending. The top of the beam is in tension and the bottom is in compression. Material at the midpoint of the longitudinal axis are not subject to either force.

The change in stiffness of the beam with an alteration in cross-sectional area is known as the 'second moment of area'. The bending stiffness of a plate is proportional to the third power of its thickness. It is linearly proportional to the Young's modulus of the material. The formula used to calculate this is:

Bending stiffness of rectangular plate: width x $(height)^3/_{12}$

The value is also called the 'second moment of inertia', which is the resistance to internal deformation of a beam.

The working length of a plate is important for its deflection with load. The working length is the unsupported portion of the plate (usually distance between the screws closest to the fracture site). Bending deformation of a plate is proportional to the square of the working length, and the bending stiffness is inversely proportional to the square of the working length.

5. F

6. D

7. G

8. G

The bending stiffness of an intermedullary nail is called the polar moment of inertia. It is calculated by: $radius^4\pi/64$ for a solid nail. For a hollow nail the polar moment of inertia is still proportional to $radius^4$, but the inner $radius^4$ is subtracted from outer $radius^4$: (outer $radius^4$ – inner $radius^4$) $\pi/4$.

A solid nail of the same areas as a hollow nail has a greater bending stiffness. By manufacturing a hollow nail rather than solid, the outer diameter can be increased for the same volume of material. This increases the stiffness while maintaining the same weight and volume of material as a solid cylinder.

The torsional stiffness of a nail is proportional to the radius[4] and the stiffness of a nail in bending is inversely proportional to the square of its working length. The torsional stiffness of a nail is inversely proportional to its working length.

9. **B**

10. **F**

11. **G**

12. **A**

13. **F**

14. **G**

According to strain theory a maximum amount of strain across a fracture site can be tolerated by the cells to allow progression of fracture healing (strain is defined as change in length over initial length). With progression of the stages of fracture healing there is a reduction in the strain across the fracture gap that allows the next phase of healing to proceed. If the strains at the fracture site exceed the maximum tolerated then healing halts and a hypertrophic non-union results. In this case progression to union may be achieved by improving stability.

The maximum tolerated strains during healing are:

Granulation tissue – 100%

Woven bone – 10%

Lamellar bone – 2%

In the case given there is no evidence of healing and therefore the strain at the fracture site is greater than 100%. After exchange of the intramedullary nail the callus appears on the radiographs. The strain is about 10% at this time. After union the fracture has healed so the lamellar bone can withstand 2% strain.

Perren S. Evolution of the internal fixation of long bone fractures J Bone Joint Surg [Br] 2002; 84–B:1093–1110.

Chapter 4

Nerve and Muscle

MCQ 20
EMQ 10

Multiple Choice Questions

1. **What is the primary function of the T-tubules found within muscle tissue?**
   a. Allow rapid access of glucose and oxygen to all parts of the fibre during contraction
   b. Form anchorage points at the site of integration between muscle tissue and collagen fibres at myotendinous junction
   c. Act as a calcium ion repository during the resting state
   d. Allow rapid propagation of action potential into the muscle fibre during contraction
   e. Act as a site for the post-synaptic breakdown and recycling of acetylcholine

2. **What is the approximate velocity of nerve impulse conduction in $A\delta$ fibres?**
   a. $10ms^{-1}$
   b. $20ms^{-1}$
   c. $50ms^{-1}$
   d. $100ms^{-1}$
   e. $500ms^{-1}$

3. **Which one of the following statements about neuron function in humans is TRUE?**

   a. The resting membrane potential is -50mV
   b. The Donnan effect refers to the equilibrium reached between leakage of potassium ions out of the cell, and those being pumped back in by the Na^+/K^+ exchange pump
   c. The refractory period describes a point at which an action potential 'jumps' past a myelinated area (between nodes of Ranvier) during saltatory conduction
   d. Although the voltage-gated potassium channels open more slowly than the sodium channels during the action potential, they close first
   e. The higher membrane leakage of potassium than sodium is the single biggest contributor to generation of the resting potential

4. **Which one of the following statements about motor units is FALSE?**

   a. A motor unit is defined as all the muscle fibres innervated by a single motor neuron
   b. A motor unit cannot be activated without causing contraction of all muscle fibres within the unit
   c. Stimulation of different motor units within a given muscle is asynchronous
   d. All nerve fibres within a single motor unit are of the same type
   e. A motor unit with a larger number of muscle fibres results in relatively poor fine control of movement

5. **Which one of the following statements regarding the structural organisation of the different elements within skeletal muscle is TRUE?**

   a. The perimysium surrounds individual muscle fibres
   b. Each myofibril is made up of several individual muscle fibres
   c. One fascicle is made up of a number of muscle fibres, each coated individually in endomysium
   d. All fibres within a given muscle are of the same type
   e. Each sarcomere is contained within a coating of endomysium

6. **Which of the following factors is NOT associated with a decrease in nerve conduction velocity?**
   a. Infancy
   b. Reduction in temperature
   c. Loss of myelin sheath
   d. More proximal location
   e. Smaller neuronal diameter

7. **Which of the following is NOT a feature of Meissner's corpuscles?**
   a. Specific sensitivity to deep pressure
   b. Unmyelinated nerve ending
   c. Innervation by Aβ nerve fibre
   d. Rapid adaptation
   e. Present in dermal papillae

8. **Which one of the following statements regarding isokinetic muscle contraction is FALSE?**
   a. Resistance varies depending on the force applied
   b. Muscle tension remains constant throughout the arc of movement
   c. Isokinetic training can only be undertaken using specialised equipment
   d. Both eccentric and concentric components occur during isokinetic contraction
   e. Isokinetic contractions are believed significantly to increase skeletal muscle blood flow

9. **Which one of the following statements concerning muscle spindles is TRUE?**
   a Their sensitivity is regulated by γ-motor neurones
   b. They initiate a bi-synaptic stretch reflex
   c. They contain extrafusal myofibres
   d. They contain a central contractile region in addition to sensory segments at each end
   e. The afferent axon from a muscle spindle terminates at a synapse in the dorsal root ganglion

10. **Which one of the following statements concerning neuromuscular transmission is FALSE?**

    a. The neuromuscular cleft measures approximately 50nm
    b. The arrival of an action potential at the end of the motor neurone causes an influx of calcium ions into the synaptic knob
    c. Acetylcholine causes an increase in the permeability of the motor end plate to calcium ions
    d. The acetylcholine receptors in the skeletal muscle motor end plate are of the nicotinic subtype
    e. The effects of acetylcholine in the synaptic cleft can be potentiated by the use of the cholinesterase inhibitor neostigmine

11. **Which one of the following statements concerning skeletal muscle injury is FALSE?**

    a. Denervation of skeletal muscle results in decreased acetylcholine sensitivity
    b. Midsubstance tears are less common than those at the myotendinous junction
    c. The scar tissue that forms following muscle belly injury typically has only 50% of the tension capacity of normal muscle tissue
    d. Early surgical repair of muscle belly lacerations has not been shown significantly to increase muscle fibre regeneration distally
    e. Partial loss of the nerve supply to a muscle eventually leads to an increase in the amplitude of recorded motor unit action potentials

12. **Which of the following modalities is transmitted in the lateral spinothalamic tract?**

    a. Ipsilateral pain sensation
    b. Contralateral motor function
    c. Ipsilateral sensation to light touch
    d. Contralateral temperature sensation
    e. Ipsilateral proprioception

13. **Which of the following is NOT a feature of the parasympathetic nervous system?**

    a. Pre-ganglionic neurotransmission via muscarinic acetylcholine receptors
    b. Arises from cranial nerves III, VII, IX, X and sacral nerves S2, S3, and S4
    c. Negative chronotropic effect
    d. Innervation of myenteric plexus
    e. Synapse between pre- and post-ganglionic fibres close to target organs

14. **In a nerve conduction study, the F-response:**

    a. Is the electronic representation of the Motor Unit Action Potential that results from motor neuron stimulation
    b. Is the electrophysiological equivalent of a stretch reflex mediated by Aα fibres
    c. Allows calculation of nerve conduction velocity between the stimulating and indifference electrodes
    d. Allows calculation of nerve conduction velocity between the stimulating and recording electrodes
    e. Results from retrograde transmission up the nerve to the anterior horn cells, followed by 'reflected' transmission back down to the recording electrode

15. **Which of the following statements regarding myosin is TRUE?**

    a. A myosin filament comprises approximately 50 individual myosin molecules
    b. The macromolecular structure of myosin incorporates numerous tropomyosin subunits
    c. Each myosin molecule comprises 2 light and 2 heavy chains
    d. Functions of the myosin head include integral ATPase activity
    e. The molecular weight of a single myosin molecule is approximately 48,000

16. **Which one of the following is NOT a feature of axonotmesis?**
    a. Wallerian degeneration
    b. Discontinuity of perineurium
    c. Discontinuity of epineurium
    d. Distortion of the myelin sheath
    e. Recovery of pain sensation before proprioception

17. **Which one of the following features is suggestive of a lower rather than upper motor neuron injury?**
    a. Absence of clonus
    b. Absence of fasciculations
    c. Preservation of muscle bulk
    d. Babinski's sign
    e. Increased tone

18. **Which one of the following is NOT a characteristic feature of Type 1 skeletal muscle fibres?**
    a. High myoglobin content
    b. High ATPase content
    c. Large number of mitochondria
    d. Extensive triglyceride stores
    e. Resistance to fatigue

19. **Which one of the following is NOT a generally accepted prerequisite for undertaking muscle/tendon transfer surgery in the hand and forearm?**
    a. The patient should be at least 4 years old
    b. The hand should be sensate
    c. The donor should be one of at least two muscles effecting the same movement
    d. The affected joint should be mobile and free of scar tissue
    e. There should be no neurological dysfunction elsewhere in the affected limb

20. **Which one of the following best describes the processes that occur in skeletal muscle during excitation-contraction coupling, following an increase in intracellular calcium concentration?**

    a. A conformational change causes tropomyosin to displace from the troponin/myosin complex, allowing engagement between actin and myosin; ATPase activity produces sliding of the myosin heads pulling myosin past the actin

    b. A conformational change causes tropomyosin to displace from the troponin/myosin complex, allowing engagement between actin and myosin; ATPase activity produces sliding of the actin heads pulling myosin past the actin

    c. A conformational change causes troponin I to displace from the tropomyosin/myosin complex, allowing engagement between actin and myosin; ATPase activity produces sliding of the myosin heads pulling myosin past the actin

    d. A conformational change causes troponin I to displace from the tropomyosin/actin complex, allowing engagement between actin and myosin; ATPase activity produces sliding of the myosin heads pulling myosin past the actin

    e. A conformational change causes troponin C to displace from the tropomyosin/actin complex, allowing engagement between actin and myosin; ATPase activity produces sliding of the myosin heads pulling myosin past the actin

Extended Matching Questions

SCENARIO I OPTIONS

A Myosin filaments
B T-tubules
C Sarcoplasmic reticulum
D Junction between sarcomeres
E Tropomyosin molecules
F Myotendinous junction

G Gap between actin filaments
H Gap between myosin filaments
I Neuromuscular junction
J Proteinaceous connection between myosin filaments

The following 5 stems all concern the appearance of skeletal muscle under light or electron microscopy. For each of the following micrographic features, select the structural component represented by that feature. Each option may be used once, more than once, or not at all.

1. A band

2. I band

3. Z disc

4. M lines

5. H bands

SCENARIO II OPTIONS

A Myosin

B Sarcolemma

C Sarcoplasmic reticulum

D T-tubules

E Tropomyosin

F Troponin I

G Troponin T

H Voltage-gated calcium channel

I Voltage-gated potassium channel

J Voltage-gated sodium channel

The following 5 stems all relate to the functional mechanisms of nerve and muscle physiology. For each stem, select the structural component primarily responsible. Each option may be used once, more than once, or not at all.

6. Responsible for repolarisation at the end of a nerve action potential

7. Comprises a phospholipid bilayer with a superimposed coating of polysaccharides and collagen fibres

8. Responsible for rapid transmission of muscle action potential from the cell membrane to the contractile structures within the central portion of the cell

9. 'Blocks' active sites on actin filaments in the resting state

10. Responsible for perpetuation of muscle action potential along the cell membrane

Answers: Chapter 4

MCQ 20
EMQ 10

Multiple Choice Answers

1. D The T- (or *transverse*) tubule system comprises a series of invaginations of the sarcolemma (cell membrane) into the main body of the muscle fibre. When depolarisation of the membrane occurs with arrival of an Action Potential (AP), this is propagated into the muscle fibre via the T-tubule system, which allows contraction throughout the fibre to occur simultaneously. This process is further facilitated by the sarcoplasmic reticulum (SR), with which the T-tubules are in continuity; the SR serves as an intracellular calcium repository.

2. B Nerve fibres fall into 3 groups – A, B or C – dependent on their diameter and function. The A fibres are a family of myelinated afferent and efferent fibres within the somatic nervous system, whose conduction velocities range from 20–120ms^{-1} (with larger fibres conducting faster). B fibres are also myelinated but with a small diameter; they are the preganglionic fibres of the autonomic nervous system. The C group entirely comprises unmyelinated fibres, and like the B group have small diameter and low conduction velocity.

These conduction velocities and primary sites of the different groups are as follows:

Type of Nerve fibre	Function	Conduction velocity (*ms⁻¹)
Aα	Efferent/afferent to muscle/muscle stretch receptors	100–120
Aβ	Linked to specific stretch receptors (eg. Pacinian corpuscle)	50
Aγ	Muscle spindle efferents (detect stretch)	20
Aδ	Pain and temperature conduction	20
B	Autonomic nervous system	10
C	Preganglionic autonomic – slow pain, thermoceptors, mechanoceptors	2

3. E Several factors contribute to generation of the normal resting potential of -70mV in human nerve tissue. The Na^+/K^+ ATPase pump pumps sodium out of, and potassium into the cell; however, the presence of permanently open potassium channels in the membrane allows leakage back out of K^+, causing a loss of positive charge inside the cell. Other factors contributing to this process include leakage into the cell of Cl^- ions, and the Donnan effect (or equilibrium), whereby charged particles, either side of a semi-permeable membrane may distribute unevenly across the two sides; this is due to the presence of large, charged, organic molecules that are unable to diffuse across the lipid bilayer.

4. A The definition of a motor unit is: one motor neuron *plus* all the muscle fibres it innervates, all of which will be of the same type (it has been experimentally shown that surgically changing the type of nerve fibre innervating the motor unit leads to a change in fibre type over a period of time). Activation of the neuron therefore always causes simultaneous contraction of all fibres in the motor unit – a larger number of muscle fibres innervated by one neuron increases the strength of contraction, but at the cost of a loss of fine control. To avoid jerkiness in contraction, motor units are recruited at slightly different times, leading to a smooth contraction.

5. C All skeletal muscles are subdivided into fascicles, each with its own perimyseal coating. The fascicle in turn contains individual muscle fibres; every fibre is surrounded by a layer of endomysium. An individual muscle fibre comprises many myofibrils, each of which is itself composed of numerous sarcomeres. Sarcomeres are composed of actin and myosin myofilaments. The muscle as a whole is surrounded by the epimysium. Although a particular muscle may tend to have a predominance of a particular fibre type, all fibre types are, to an extent, represented in every muscle.

Skeletal muscle in decreasing hierarchy:

Epimysium = connective tissue sheath surrounding the whole muscle

Perimysium = white fibrous and areolar connective tissue surrounding each fascicle

Fascicle = bundle of skeletal muscle fibres

Endomysium = areolar connective tissue surrounding each muscle fibre

Muscle Fibre (Myofibre) = a muscle cell

Myofibrils = contractile protein organelles

Myofilaments = composed of chains of sarcomeres composed of:

- thick filaments – made of myosin
- thin filaments – made of actin

6. D Both the amplitude and velocity of neuronal conduction are affected by a number of factors, as follows:

- Conduction velocity is reduced at extremes of age
- Nerve conduction is faster in the upper limb than lower, and within a given limb is slower at more distal sites
- Larger nerve diameter leads to faster conduction
- Loss of myelination reduces speed of conduction
- Hypothermia significantly reduces conduction

7. A The four main types of mechanoreceptor nerve ending (corpuscle) found in the skin are:

- Meissner's – light touch
- Pacinian – flutter
- Ruffini – vibration
- Merkel – deep steady pressure

All are innervated by Aβ fibres; in addition there are *free endings* (innervated by Aδ fibres) which are responsive to mechanical, thermal and noxious stimuli. Meissner's corpuscles are rapidly adaptive – they sense *change* in pressure more than pressure itself. The dermal papillae are small projections of the dermis up into the epidermis, which contain high numbers of nerve endings.

8. B There are three main types of muscle contraction:

- Isometric – the length of the muscle remains constant whilst tension (force) changes
- Isotonic – tension (force applied) is constant whilst length changes
- Isokinetic – velocity of muscle contraction is constant; resistance varies with force applied.

Within each of these, both concentric and eccentric contraction may occur (contraction with reduction or increase in length, respectively). Isokinetic training can only be undertaken using special equipment, but is believed to result in significant improvements in blood flow, strength and endurance.

9. A The muscle stretch reflex is a typical mono-synaptic spinal reflex, and has a central role in the control of both muscle tone and posture. The muscle spindle is the stretch receptor for this reflex, and comprises a central receptor region inbetween two contractile regions, which contain intrafusal fibres innervated by Aγ- motor neurones from the ventral horn in the spinal cord. By altering the tone (and therefore length) of the contractile regions, this adjusts the sensitivity of the spindle. The Aγ- motor neurones are also co-activated during normal muscle contraction (which is innervated by Aγ- motor neurones) to prevent a negative feedback loop from inhibiting further contraction.

When the spindle is stretched, the spindle fires and the nerve impulse is transmitted back along the sensory neurone; this passes through the dorsal root ganglion, where the nerve has its cell body, but does not synapse here. It travels in the dorsal spinal nerve into the spinal cord, where it terminates in an excitatory synapse with the Aα- motor neurone; this increases tone in the muscle to counteract the stretch. At the same time, inhibition of the Aα- motor neurone supplying the antagonistic muscle occurs.

10. C Motor neurones terminate in an unmyelinated region known as the synaptic knob; this region holds numerous vesicles containing the neuromtransmitter acetylcholine (ACh). The arrival of an action potential increases the permeability of the presynaptic membrane to calcium ions, as a result of which there is a large influx, which in turn causes ACh to be released into the synaptic cleft (50nm across). The ACh rapidly diffuses across the cleft to bind to receptors on the motor end plate; a local end-plate potential (EPP) is established by a change in membrane permeability to sodium and potassium.

This EPP in turn leads to an action potential in the surrounding muscle (due to calcium influx) and the muscle contracts. Once the ACh has been released from the receptor, cholinesterases in the cleft then break it down; a process that can be inhibited by several pharmacological agents including neostigmine. In the autonomic nervous system there are noradrenaline receptors as well as both nicotinic and muscarinic ACh receptors; however, in skeletal muscle all ACh receptors are of the nicotinic subtype.

11.   A   A number of mechanisms may lead to muscle injury, but in all cases the effect is potentiated by the release of intracellular calcium, which activates a number of destructive enzymes. Muscle belly laceration results in rapid wasting distally, which is permanent unless reinnervation occurs. However, surgical repair has not been shown to confer any significant advantage in terms of distal fibre regeneration, and at best only 50% recovery of pre-injury strength can be expected following complete muscle belly transection.

Denervation (lower motor neurone injury) leads to atrophy, fibrillation and increased acetylcholine sensitivity. Over a period of time, reinnervation of the muscle may occur; but following this, or after partial denervation, the size of the motor units increases, which leads to increased amplitude of the motor unit action potential.

12.   D   The key somatic modalities transmitted in the spinal cord are arranged as follows:

Afferent	
Dorsal columns (ipsilateral)	Deep touch, proprioception, vibration
Lateral spinothalamic (contralateral)	Pain and temperature
Anterior spinothalamic (contralateral)	Light touch
Efferent	
Lateral corticospinal (contralateral)	Motor
Lateral corticospinal (ipsilateral)	Motor

13.   A   The autonomic nervous system is subdivided into the sympathetic (SNS) – 'flight, fight, fright' – and parasympathetic (PSNS) nervous systems. In both systems, the pre-ganglionic neurotransmission is via the nicotinic ACh receptor; in the PSNS, post-synaptic transmission is via the muscarinic ACh receptor (in the SNS the post-ganglionic neurotransmitter is noradrenaline).

Parasympathetic innervation is carried in the oculomotor, facial, glossopharyngeal and vagus nerves; as well as the S2–S4 nerve roots. In simple terms, the physiological effects of the PSNS are to reduce blood pressure and pulse rate, and to potentiate the functioning of the gastrointestinal tract via the myenteric plexus. Unlike the SNS, whose synapses are in the sympathetic chain, and whose post-ganglionic fibres are long, the synapses in the PSNS tend to be close to the relevant target organs.

14. E Nerve conduction studies are recorded by measurement of latency, waveform and amplitude of an impulse in a recording electrode, following initiation of an action potential by a stimulating electrode. Velocity can be calculated from the distance and latency together. A ground electrode in the target muscle can also measure motor unit action potentials – the timing of this measurement provides information about synaptic function, whilst the amplitude is a measure of the number of motor units recruited.

In addition to the main recorded nerve impulse, the sensory electrode may also record the *H-reflex* and *F-response*. The H-reflex results from stimulation of afferent Aα fibres which synapse in the dorsal horn causing a stretch-reflex-like impulse to be transmitted back down to the recording electrode via motor neurons. Conversely, the F-response is the equivalent of an 'echo'; retrograde impulse transmission up the motor neuron then 'bounces' back down to the recording electrode.

15. D Myosin is one of the two main contractile filaments within muscle (the other being actin). Each myosin filament comprises at least 200 individual molecules; each of these comprises 2 heavy and 4 light chains, and has a molecular weight of roughly 480,000. The ATPase activity of the myosin head is integral to its function – cleavage of ATP provides the energy necessary for the head to 'spin' and thus pull the myosin and actin past one another. Tropomyosin is a separate molecule, which is intimately related to actin; in the resting state it blocks the active sites on the actin molecule.

16. C In axonotmesis there is disruption of the axon (and myelin sheath), but not the epineurium and perineurium. In neuronotmesis all elements of the nerve are disrupted. Both axonotmesis and neuronotmesis result in Wallerian degeneration (a breakdown of axons and myelin to provide clean endoneuronal tubes for sprouting axons). The axons enlarge into a stump and then sprout within about 96 hours – only in neurapraxia does this not occur. Pain is the first modality to recover following nerve injury.

17. A Both upper (UMN) and lower motor neurone (LMN) lesions are associated with a reduction in power. However, a number of clinical features allow differentiation between the two:

Feature	UMN	LMN
Tone	↑	↓
Power	↓	↓
Reflexes	↑	↓
Muscle atrophy	–	✓
Babinski's sign (upgoing plantar response)	✓	–
Muscle fasciculations	–	✓
Clonus	✓	–

18. B All skeletal muscles have a combination of type I ('slow twitch') and type 2 ('fast twitch') fibres, although certain activities such as athletic training can lead to a predominance of one over the other. Type 2 can be further subdivided into types 2a and 2b. The features are summarised below; the mnemonic 'Slow Red Ox' for type 1 fibres is a useful *aide-memoire*.

Type 1
- Red
- Oxidative
- Large amount of myoglobin
- High triglyceride content
- Numerous mitochondria
- Low ATPase levels
- Require O_2 for sustained activity
- Fatigue-resistant

Type 2a
- White
- Both oxidative and glycolytic
- Resist fatigue
- Numerous mitochondria

Type 2b

- White
- Glycolytic
- Anaerobic
- Low triglyceride content
- Sparse mitochondria
- High ATPase levels
- Quickly fatigue

19. E The principles of tendon transfer surgery can be remembered as the 'Eight S's':

- $\underline{S}$ensible patient
- $\underline{S}$ufficient age (normally considered to be >4)
- $\underline{S}$ensate hand
- $\underline{S}$carfree tissue
- $\underline{S}$upple joint
- $\underline{S}$acrificable donors (i.e. at least one other muscle should effect the same activity)
- $\underline{S}$ingle action
- $\underline{S}$traight line of pull

Neurological dysfunction elsewhere in the limb is not a contra-indication provided it does not impinge on the criteria listed above.

20. D The mechanisms of excitation-contraction coupling are frequently asked in both written and oral examinations. The cellular influx of Ca^{2+} causes conformational changes in the troponin complex (subunits C, I and T) by binding to Troponin C. In the resting state, the conformation of the tropomyosin/actin complex is such that the active sites on the actin are covered; the conformational change in the troponins displaces the tropomyosin from these active sites allowing interaction between actin and the myosin heads. ATPase activity in the myosin head causes conformational change in the head such that it rotates, pulling the myosin and actin past one another. As they uncouple from one another ADP is released, the calcium dissociates from the troponin complex and is actively pumped back into the T-tubules and sarcoplasmic reticulum.

Individual troponin subunits serve different functions:

- Troponin C binds to calcium ions to produce a conformational change in Troponin I
- Troponin T binds to tropomyosin to form a troponin-tropomyosin complex
- Troponin I binds to actin to hold the troponin-tropomyosin complex in place

Extending Matching Answers

1. **A**
2. **H**
3. **D**
4. **J**
5. **G**

The radiographic bands visible microscopically within the sarcomere are regularly asked within all sections of most postgraduate orthopaedic examinations, so are worth committing to memory. These bands represent the following structures:

- **A bands** (*anisotropic*) – myosin filaments
- **I bands** (*isotropic*) – gap between A bands containing actin filaments bridging sarcomeres
- **Z discs** (*zwischen; 'between'*) – between sarcomeres
- **H bands** (*heller; 'bright'*) – myosin only, between actin filaments
- **M lines** (*Mittel; 'middle'*) – site of M-band protein connection between adjacent myosin filaments

6. **I**
7. **B**
8. **D**
9. **E**
10. **H**

The two chief contractile elements within the myofibril are *actin* and *myosin*. In the resting state, the active sites on actin are 'blocked' by tropomyosin, which is complexed with the actin, and is also closely associated with complexes of the troponin C, I and T. Acetylcholine crossing the synaptic cleft binds receptors on the motor end plate; this leads to a local influx of sodium ions, and the resultant depolarisation opens voltage-gated calcium channels which then transmit the muscle action potential along the sarcolemma (the cell wall, formed of a true membrane closely associated with a polysaccharide 'wall' also containing numerous collagen fibres).

The T-tubule system transmits the action potential into the cell and further calcium ions are released into the cytoplasm from the sarcoplasmic reticulum. This causes a conformational change in the troponins such that tropomyosin is 'pulled off' the actin, which then binds to the myosin heads. Rotation of the head (an energy-dependent process requiring cleavage of ATP) pulls the myosin and actin past one another. As they uncouple from one another ADP is released, the calcium dissociates from the troponin complex and is actively pumped back into the T-tubules and sarcoplasmic reticulum.

The action potential in a nerve results from the opening of voltage-gated sodium channels; these rapidly close, at about the same time as slower voltage-gated potassium channels open to allow repolarisation. The time delay in this process accounts for the *latent period* between action potentials.

Chapter 5

Connective Tissue

MCQ 24
EMQ 10

Multiple Choice Questions

1. **Which of the following is the best answer regarding the structure of collagen?**

    a. Type 1 collagen has 4 chains
    b. The orientation of proteoglycans contributes to anisotropy in lamellar bone
    c. The associated proteoglycans have a polysaccharide core
    d. Type 2 collagen is the predominant organic component of bone
    e. Type I collagen contains a significant proportion of glycine

2. **Which of the following is the most accurate statement about articular cartilage?**

    a. It undergoes mainly aerobic metabolism with nutrients from the sub-chondral bone
    b. Repair to injuries occurs with deposition of type 1 collagen
    c. Type X collagen is found in the deep layer
    d. Large round chondrocytes are found in the superficial layer
    e. 70% of the collagen is type 2 collagen

3. **Which of the following statements is FALSE about articular cartilage?**
   a. The superficial layer accounts for up to 20% of the depth
   b. The middle layer accounts for between 40 and 60% of the depth
   c. The deep layer accounts for approximately 30% of the depth
   d. Fibres in the deep layer are orientated perpendicular to the joint surface
   e. Water content increases with the depth of cartilage

4. **The cartilage in osteoarthritic joints differs from that in normal aging by having:**
   a. Increased water content
   b. Decreased proteoglycan degradation
   c. Increased Young's modulus
   d. Increased keratin sulphate
   e. Decreased chondrotin sulphate

5. **Which one of the following zones of articular cartilage has the highest concentration of proteoglycans?**
   a. Calcified layer
   b. Tidemark
   c. Deep
   d. Transitional/middle
   e. Superficial

6. **Which one of the following statements regarding articular cartilage is FALSE?**
   a. Cartilage responds to injury only if it passes through the tidemark
   b. The superficial layer is specialised for shear resistance
   c. Cartilage is anisotropic
   d. Type X collagen is found in the deep layer
   e. The water content of cartilage is approximately 60–80%

7. **What is the function of the type A synoviocyte?**
   a. Antigen presentation
   b. Synovial fluid production
   c. Proteoglycan degradation
   d. Hyaluronic acid production
   e. Acts as a precursor to type B synoviocytes

8. **Which one of the following processes occurs in age-related disc degeneration?**
   a. Increase in water content of the nucleus pulposus
   b. Decreased keratan sulphate:chondroitin sulphate ratio
   c. Decreased cell synthetic activity
   d. Increased concentration of blood vessels
   e. Decreased degradative enzyme activity

9. **Immobilisation of a synovial joint is NOT associated with which one of the following changes?**
   a. Thinning of the articular cartilage
   b. Softening of the articular cartilage
   c. Increase in proteoglycan concentration
   d. Decreased stiffness of associated ligaments
   e. Decreased strength of associated ligaments

10. **During the stance phase of gait which of the following is NOT thought to contribute significantly to lubrication in the hip joint?**
    a. Elastohydrodynamic (fluid film) lubrication
    b. Weeping lubrication
    c. Boosted lubrication
    d. Hydrodynamic lubrication
    e. Boundary lubrication

11. **Which one of the following statements is FALSE about the process of osteoarthritis around synovial joints?**
    a. Osteophytes are often covered in hyaline cartilage
    b. Remodelling of bone observes Wolff's law
    c. Proteoglycans are non-aggregated
    d. Chondrocytes are less metabolically active
    e. The stiffness and tensile strength of type II collagen in the articular cartilage decreases

12. **Which of the following is FALSE about the structure of the meniscus?**
    a. The predominant cell is the chondrocyte
    b. Type I collagen is the predominant collagen subtype
    c. 60–70% dry weight is composed of extracellular matrix
    d. The outer region of meniscus has a greater capacity for healing than the inner portion
    e. With aging the mechanical properties in the normal meniscus remain constant

13. **Which of the following patterns of cell changes occur in the synovium in rheumatoid arthritis?**
    a. Increase in type A and type B synoviocytes and decrease in T lymphocytes
    b. Increase in type A and type B synoviocytes and T lymphocytes
    c. Increase in type A synoviocytes with a decrease in type B and T lymphocytes
    d. Decrease in type A and B synoviocytes and an increase in T lymphocytes
    e. A decrease in all cell types

14. **Which of the following statements is FALSE about the formation and aging of the intervertebral disc?**
    a. The nucleus pulposus is derived from the notochord
    b. The anulus fibrosus is derived from mesoderm
    c. Collagen deposition in the nucleus pulposus increases with age
    d. Prolonged heavy lifting accelerates disc degeneration
    e. Smoking has a protective effect upon degenerative disc disease

15. **Which one of the following is NOT true about the mechanical properties of meniscus?**
    a. The deep layer of meniscus has circumferential fibres
    b. Fluid flow through the meniscus contributes to shock absorption
    c. Meniscal mechanical properties do not depend upon the direction of testing
    d. The orientation of the collagen fibres in the superficial layer of meniscus is random
    e. The mechanical properties of the meniscus are inhomogeneous

16. **Which one of the following is INCORRECT regarding the annulus fibrosus?**

    a. The outer layer is composed of type I collagen
    b. Functionally it has high tensile strength
    c. Collagen fibres insert directly via Sharpey's fibres into vertebral bodies
    d. The highest concentration of pyridinoline cross links are in the annulus
    e. Nerve fibres pass all the way through the disc into the nucleus pulposus

17. **Which one of the following is INCORRECT regarding the nucleus pulposus?**

    a. It has a high concentration of type II collagen
    b. It functions to resist compressive loads
    c. Nutrition of the nucleus is derived down a diffusion gradient
    d. There is a high composition of type VII collagen in the nucleus pulposus
    e. Up to 50% of the nucleus pulposus is composed of proteogly-cans in a child

18. **In which of the following positions is intradiscal pressure the highest?**

    a. Lying down
    b. Standing up
    c. Sitting
    d. Sitting forwards
    e. Reclining

19. **Which one of the following is FALSE about the properties of synovial fluid?**

    a. It displays Newtonian characteristics
    b. It contains hyaluronic acid
    c. It is produced by type B synoviocytes
    d. It is produced by the ultrafiltation of plasma
    e. It exhibits thixotropic properties

20. **Which one of the following statements regarding the meniscus is FALSE?**

    a. Only the anterior horns of the medial and lateral menisci are connected by the intermensical ligament

    b. The meniscofemoral ligaments run from the lateral meniscus to the lateral femoral condyle

    c. Medial meniscus is less mobile

    d. Both menisci receive a peripheral nerve and blood supply

    e. Mechanoreceptors have been identified in the periphery of the menisci

21. **Which one of the following statements about the damaged meniscus is FALSE?**

    a. Partial medial menisectomy increases joint loads

    b. Disruption of the intermeniscal ligament increases peak tibial stress during flexion

    c. The best results following meniscus repair occur in conjunction with ACL reconstruction

    d. Partial meniscectomy for complete posterior medial meniscus root tear is correlated with early osteoarthritis

    e. Horizontal sutures in a meniscal repair are stronger than vertical ones

22. **Regarding the menisci and the effect of tears, which one of the following statements is TRUE?**

    a. Hoop stresses in the axially loaded meniscus occur in the radially orientated fibres

    b. Radial split tears of the medial meniscus significantly increase tibiofemoral joint pressures

    c. Vertical tears of the medial meniscus do not significantly increase tibiofemoral joint pressures

    d. Repair of vertical tears does not alter the contact pressure compared with the torn meniscus

    e. Vertical tears of the medial meniscus significantly increase tibiofemoral joint pressures

23. **Which one of the following statements about the structure or function of proteoglycans is FALSE?**

   a. Proteoglycans consist of a glycosaminoglycan core and one or more branching protein chains
   b. Proteoglycans are negatively charged
   c. Hyaluronic acid is a glycosaminoglycan found in articular cartilage
   d. Aggrecans are proteoglycans that associate with hyaluronic acid to form proteoglycan aggregates
   e. The concentration of proteoglycans varies with site in the cartilage

24. **Which one of the following changes does not occur in the aging disc?**

   a. Decreased water content
   b. Increased proteoglycan concentration
   c. Increased degradative enzyme concentration
   d. Loss of disc height
   e. The cartilaginous end plates change from hyaline to calcified cartilage

Extended Matching Questions

SCENARIO I OPTIONS

A Type I   **E** Type VI

B Type II   **F** Type X

C Type III   **G** Type XIII

D Type IV

Which type of collagen listed above best fits the definition in each question below? Each option may be used once, more than once or not at all.

1. The type of collagen which is defective in osteogenesis imperfecta.

2. The major constituent of articular cartilage.

3. This collagen subtype is virtually unique to intervertebral disc.

4. This type of collagen is found in high concentrations in proliferative Dupuytren's disease.

5. This type of collagen is found in the mineralised zone of articular cartilage and is critical in mineralisation.

SCENARIO II OPTIONS

A 50%   E 180%
B 70%   F 200%
C 95%   G 300%
D 140%

Which of the responses above is the most appropriate for each of the following questions? Each option may be used once, more than once or not at all.

6. What is the percentage of medial compartmental force that passes though the intact medial meniscus in a normal knee when standing upright?

7. What is the percentage of lateral compartmental force that passes though the intact lateral meniscus in a normal knee when standing upright?

8. What is the approximate increase in the peak contact stress in the medial compartment of the tibiofemoral joint after 50% of the medial meniscus has been resected?

9. What is the approximate increase in the stress in the ACL after medial menisectomy?

10. What percentage of patients playing high level sports with a chronically ACL deficient knee will end up with a meniscal injury?

Answers: Chapter 5

MCQ 24
EMQ 10

Multiple Choice Answers

1. E The general structure of a Type I collagen molecule is one of three chains (alpha chains). Each chain possesses a characteristic tri-aminoacid sequence where every third residue is glycine, and with the other amino acids frequently represented by proline and hydroxyproline. The amino acids are coiled in a left handed helix forming an alpha chain. Three alpha chains form a larger collagen molecule. This typically involves two identical chains (alpha 1) and one different chain (alpha 2). Each alpha chain is approximately 1050 residues in length. The three chains come together to form a right-handed superhelix.

The superhelix has a macro-structure resembling a rod, with a diameter of approximately 1.5 nm and length of 300 nm. Collagen chains contribute to the tensile strength of bone, whereas the mineral phase resists compressive stress. The orientation of the collagen fibres is reported to be responsible, in part, for the anisotropy of bone. This means that bone has a different Young's modulus when loaded in the transverse versus a perpendicular manner. Bones with a predominance of collagen fibres orientated in the longitudinal axis of the bone have a greater tensional strength than those with collagen orientated in a predominantly transverse orientation.

Type 2 collagen is the predominant organic component of articular cartilage and proteoglycans are formed of glycosaminoglycans (GAGs) covalently attached to a core protein, not a polysaccharide core.

2. **B** Synovial fluid provides nutrition to articular cartilage. Repair to cartilage occurs by type 1 collagen only if the defect is full thickness, otherwise repair does not occur. Flat chondrocytes are found in the superficial layer, deep chondrocytes are round. Collagen contributes 60% of the dry weight. Collagen types II, VI, IX and XI are predominant. The main collagen in articular cartilage is type II accounting for 90–95% of the collagen. Types II, IX and XI form a mesh which serves to trap proteoglycans and provide the stiffness and strength. Type VI collagen is associated with chondrocytes to aid their attachment to the matrix. Type X collagen is associated with calcification and therefore found in the calcified cartilage layer.

3. **E** The superficial layer accounts for 10–20% of the depth of cartilage, the middle 40–60% and the deep 30%. The fibres in the superficial layer are parallel to the joint surface and are therefore good at resisting shear. The superficial layer is composed of two layers; the thinnest, most superficial layer is called the 'lamina splendens' which is acellular. This layer functions to resist shear and prevent leakage of proteoglycans. Still in the superficial layer, but deep to lamina splendens, flattened chondrocytes are arranged parallel to the articular surface. There is a higher concentration of collagen and water than proteoglycan in this layer. With increasing depth the concentration of proteoglycans increases and the water concentration decreases. The collagen concentration also decreases with increasing depth.

The middle layer has the fibres orientated in an oblique manner and crossing, in a transition from parallel to perpendicular. By contrast the deep fibres are perpendicular to the joint surface to resist compression.

The tide mark zone is the junction between the deep and calcified zones and is visible as a basophilic line when stained histologically. The calcified zone is a thin zone that separates the deep zone from the subchondral bone.

4. **A** The age related and degenerative changes occurring in articular cartilage are summarised below:

Component	Osteoarthritis-related changes	Age-related changes
Water content	Increased	Decreased
Overall effect upon collagen	Increased with more disordered matrix	No effect
Overall concentration of proteoglycans	Decreased	Decreased
Synthesis of proteoglycans	Increased	No effect
Degradation of proteoglycans	Increased	Decreased
Young's modulus	Decreased	Increased
Concentation of chondroitin sulphate	Increased	Decreased
Concentation of karatan sulphate	Decreased	Increased
Numbers of chondrocytes	No effect	Decreased

5. **C** The deep zone of articular cartilage has the highest concentration of proteoglycans. The proteoglycan concentration increases and water concentration decreases from superficial to deep zones. Water concentration decreases despite a rise in hydrophilic proteoglycans due to an increased density in the matrix.

6. **D** Cartilage has both viscoelastic and anisotropic properties. The orientation of the collagen fibrils in the superficial layer, parallel to the joint surface, makes it the layer most resistant to shear. Injuries to cartilage will only heal by type I collagen deposition if the injury passes through the tidemark zone.

Type X collagen is only found associated with bone mineralisation, and not the deep layer of cartilage. The water content of articular cartilage is about 70%.

7. A Type A synoviocyte has phagocytic functions, and can be considered similar functionally to a macrophage (it is derived from blood monocytes and has an antigen presenting role). Synovial fluid is made by the type B synoviocyte. The function of the type C synoviocyte is unknown.

8. C The following processes are found in age related disc degeneration:

- In the nucleus pulposus there is an increase in proteoglycans, a decrease in water content and a reduction in the number of cells. There is no change in the amount of collagen.
- In the annulus fibrosus there is an increased incidence of cartilage cracks and tears.
- There is an increase in the keratan sulphate:chondroitin sulphate ratio.
- There is a decrease in the concentration of blood vessels in the end plate and the amount of nutrition delivered to the disc.

9. C Joint immobilisation has detrimental effects upon the articular cartilage and ligaments. The cartilage softens and thins with an associated decrease in proteoglycan concentration. The ligaments become less stiff and strong. The ligaments can recover back to their pre-immobilisation mechanical characteristics, but the loss in mechanical properties is much quicker than the time taken to regain them.

10. A All types of lubrication occur in synovial joints during walking. During with swing phase when loads through the hip are the lowest and the fluid film is thick, fluid film lubrication is thought to occur. As the cartilage elastically deforms, the asperities are smoothed out and therefore elastohydrodynamic lubrication is thought to occur. When the joint is loaded the fluid is squeezed out and boundary lubrication is thought to predominate. With longer periods of standing there is likely to be a greater contribution of fluid changes within and from the cartilage, weeping and boosted lubrication.

11. D Osteophytes have both bony and cartilaginous portions, with the majority being covered with normal hyaline cartilage. In OA the bone is remodelled in a normal manner with trabeculae being laid down according to Wolff's law, whereby trabeculae are laid down parallel to lines of stress applied to the bone.

The articular cartilage contains less well ordered collagen which is less stiff, and proteoglycans are non-aggregated and of a lower concentration than in normal cartilage with the loss of proteoglycan being related to the severity of the disease. However, the chondrocytes are more metabolically active.

See table in feedback to question 4.

12. A The predominant cell type in the meniscus is the fibrochondrocyte. They synthesize a large amount of type I collagen and lower, but significant amounts of type II collagen and aggrecan.

Type I collagen is the predominant collagen, orientated into radial and longitudinal fibres to dissipate the applied stresses. The outer portion (approximately 25%) in the adult is vascularised and has a greater capacity for healing. The mechanical properties of the normal meniscus do not alter greatly with age.

13. B The most abundant cell populations in rheumatoid arthritis are type A and B synoviocytes, and infiltration of the synovium with T lymphocytes is also seen. Other cells that are thought to have a role in the disease are B lymphocytes, plasma cells, dendritic cells, mast cells and osteoclasts.

14. E In the aging disc, water content, proteoglycan content, size, and concentration are decreased, and keratan sulfate and collagen content are increased.

The anulus fibrosus is derived from mesoderm and is divided into outer and inner layers. The nucleus pulposus is derived from the primitive notochord, with the primary function of resisting compressive loads. The two structures are distinct in the infant but with age they become less so as the disc dehydrates and the collagen blends. A reversal of the orientation of the inner layers of the anulus fibrosus is seen to occur, so that rather than bulging outwards, the inner fibres of the anulus bulge inwards. Nutrition for the disc comes from the vascular plexus in the end plate and anything disrupting this, such as smoking, can lead to accelerated disc degeneration.

15. C Over 90% of meniscal tissue is composed of type I collagen.

The orientation of collagen fibres changes with progression through the meniscus:
- Superficial layer has mainly random orientation
- Middle layer is composed of a random orientation with some radial fibres
- Deep layer has mainly circumferential orientation of fibres with radial fibres

Glycosaminoglycans are up to 2% of the weight of the meniscus and are held within the collagen fibres. The mechanical properties therefore are dependent upon fluid flow though a porous material and then a later deformation of the meniscal tissue. The combination of fluid flow and orientation of the collagen makes the mechanical properties of the meniscus both anisotropic and inhomogeneous.

16. E The primary components of the disc are collagen, water, and proteoglycans. The annulus is composed of an outer layer of type I collagen and an inner layer of type II collagen giving the annulus its tensile strength. The outer layer fibres run obliquely and insert directly into the vertebral body via Sharpey's fibres. These fibres run perpendicular to one another and resist movement in multiple planes.

All of the collagen fibrils are highly crosslinked with pyridinoline residues. Nerve fibres innervate the outer but not the inner layer of the annulus, terminating before the nucleus pulposus.

17. D The primary function of the nucleus pulposus is to resist compressive loads. It has a high concentration of type II collagen and proteoglycans.

Nutrients to the nucleus diffuse down a concentration gradient from the anulus and endplate, a process which is concentration and charge dependent. There is a high content (up to 20% in the nucleus) of type VI collagen and up to 50% of the nucleus consists of proteoglycans in a child, a concentration that decreases with aging.

18. D Compared with pressure in the upright standing position, reclining reduces the pressure by 50–80%, unsupported sitting increases the load by 40%, leaning forward by over 100%, and the position of forward flexion and rotation by 400%.

(Nachemson et al. Spine 1981, Vol 6, Issue 1)

19. **A** Synovial fluid is an ultra-filtrate of plasma plus lubricin, hyaluronic acid, glycoproteins and degradative enzymes produced by type B synoviocytes. Due to hydrogen bonds formed between water and these large molecules, synovial fluid has non-Newtonian fluid behaviour; meaning that its viscosity is not constant and in the case of synovial fluid, is inversely related to shear rate. The relationship between shear rate and viscosity is determined by the orientation of the hyaluronic acid molecules as the fluid is sheared. This behaviour is termed thixotropic and can be described as "shear thinning"; the longer the shear stress is applied, the lower the viscosity.

20. **B** The intermeniscal ligament connects the anterior horns of the medial and lateral meniscus. The meniscofemoral ligaments of Humphrey and Wrisberg run anterior and posterior to the PCL respectively. They connect the lateral meniscus to the medial femoral condyle. The medial meniscus is attached around its periphery and is therefore more stable than the lateral which has a hiatus for popliteus. Both menisci receive a peripheral blood and nerve supply. Mechanoreceptors have been shown to be numerous around the periphery and in the anterior and posterior horns of the meniscus.

21. **E** Partial medial menisectomy increases joint loads and if the root is partially excised there is an associated risk of early arthritis. Meniscal repair in a mechanically abnormal knee is likely to fail and therefore should be carried out at the same time as ligament reconstruction. Good results have been reported for meniscal repair in conjunction with ACL reconstruction.

Barber *et al.* reported successful meniscal healing occurred in 92% of repairs performed with ACL reconstructions, but only in 67% of meniscal repairs performed in ACL-deficient knees.

Release of the anterior intermeniscal ligament increases joint contact pressures during flexion, with the largest change at 40 degrees of flexion (Paci *et al.*), and vertical sutures are biomechanically stronger than horizontal ones. (Rankin *et al.*)

Barber FA, Click SD. Meniscus repair rehabilitation with concurrent anterior cruciate reconstruction. Arthroscopy 1997 Aug;13(4):433–7.

Paci JM. et al. Knee medial compartment contact pressure increases with release of the type I anterior intermeniscal ligament. Am. J Sports Med. 2009 Jul;37(7):1412–6. Epub 2009 Mar 13.

Rankin C. et al. A Biomechanical Analysis of Meniscal Repair Techniques. Am J Sports Med July 2002 vol. 30 no. 4 492–497.

22. **E** Hoop stresses in the axially loaded meniscus occur in the circumferential fibres, not radial ones. In a cadaveric study of meniscal tears, Muriuki *et al.* demonstrated that:

- Radial split tears of the medial meniscus do not significantly change in tibiofemoral joint contact pressures.
- Vertical tears of the medial meniscus significantly increase tibiofemoral joint contact pressure in line with those associated with total medial meniscectomy.
- Repair of the vertical tear, in general, restored contact pressures to normal.

Muriuki MG et al. Changes in tibiofemoral contact mechanics following radial split and vertical tears of the medial meniscus an in vitro investigation of the efficacy of arthroscopic repair. JBJS Am. 2011 Jun 15;93(12):1089–95.

23. **A** A proteoglycan is composed of a protein core with gylcosaminoglycan (GAG) polysaccharide side chains. Side chains include chondroitin sulphate and keratan sulphate (all GAGs). Hyaluronic acid differs from other GAGs because it is not found as a proteoglycan.

Approximately 10% of the proteoglycan is protein and 90% are GAGs. The proteoglycans are negatively changed. Aggrecan is the commonest proteoglycan. It is a large proteoglycan consisting of a protein core with chondroitin sulphate and keratan suphate side chains.

24. **B** With aging there is decreased water content, decreased proteoglycan concentration, an increase in the degradative enzyme concentration, but no change in absolute collagen content. There is also loss of disc height and gradual calcification of the end plate of the disc.

Extending Matching Answers

1.   A   Osteogenesis imperfecta is secondary to a defective production of type I collagen. It is usually due to a substitution of larger amino acids into the glycine position in the collagen chain. This substitution prevents close packing of the collagen and leads to macroscopic problems with the material properties of collagen.

2.   B   Type II collagen is the major collagen component of articular cartilage and hyaline cartilage. Its main function is to provide tensile strength and three dimensional stability to the tissue. Bound proteoglycans are responsible for the surface and hydrophilic properties of articular cartilage.

3.   E   Type VI collagen is found in high concentrations in the intervertebral disc, along with type I and type II collagen. It has been reported to perform an "anchoring function" apparently and does not function as a covalently crosslinked structural polymer.

4.   C   Type III collagen is found in immature scar tissue, in the tissue found in the proliferative phase of Dupuytren's disease and in immature woven bone/ fracture callus

5.   F   Type X collagen is found in the mineralised zone of articular cartilage and hypertrophic cartilage.

6.   A   See answer 8.

7.   B   See answer 8.

8. **A**   The meniscus distributes the loads across the knee and acts as a shock absorber. The medial meniscus transmits up to 50% of the applied load in the medial compartment, and the lateral meniscus transmits up to 70% of the applied load in the lateral compartment of the knee.

The menisci transmit loads of up to 1470 N and cover up to 71% of the contact surface area around the periphery of the tibial plateau. If a partial or total menisectomy is performed then there is a change in the contact pressures in the knee. A 50% medial menisectomy reportedly increases peak contact stress by 43% when compared with an intact knee. The increases with increasing degrees of meniscal resection are: 95% (75% meniscectomy), 123% (segmental meniscectomy), and 136% (total meniscectomy). Baratz *et al.* reported that meniscectomy leads to a 75% reduction in tibiofemoral contact area and between 200 and 300% increase in peak local contact pressures.

Lee SJ, Aadalen KJ, Malaviya P, Lorenz EP, Hayden JK, Farr J, Kang RW, Cole BJ. Am J Sports Med. 2006 Aug;34(8):1334–44.

Baratz ME, Fu FH, Mengato R. Meniscal tears: the effect of meniscectomy and of repair on intraarticular contact areas and stress in the human knee. A preliminary report. Am J Sports Med. 1986 Jul-Aug; 14(4):270–5.

McDermott ID, Amis AA. The consequences of meniscectomy. JBJS Br 2006 Dec; 88(12):1549–56.

Kurosawa H, Fukubayashi T, Nakajima H. Load-bearing mode of the knee joint: physical behavior of the knee joint with or without menisci. Clin Orthop Relat Res. 1980 Jun;(149):283–90.

9. **A**   Medial meniscectomy increases the stress across the ACL by 50% due to loss in the secondary restraint the posterior horn of the medial meniscus plays in stabilising the AP translation of the tibiofemoral joint. Vice versa, the stress on the medial meniscus increases significantly in the ACL deficient knee.

Papageorgiou et al. Am J Sports Med 2001, 29, 2, 226–231

Allen et al. Journal of Orthopaedic Research 18, 1, 109–115

10. **C**   95% of patients with ACL deficient knees who return to high-level activity will have meniscal and cartilage damage with resultant progressive arthritis.

Nebelung W, Arthroscopy 2005; 21:696

Chapter 6

Pharmacology, Inflammation and Infection

MCQ 29
EMQ 6

Multiple Choice Questions

1. Which of the following is the mode of action by which erythromycin works?

    a. Inhibition of transpeptidase enzyme
    b. Increase in cell membrane permeability
    c. Ribosomal inhibitor
    d. Interference with DNA metabolism
    e. Acts as an antimetabolite

2. Which of the following antibiotics is associated with tendon rupture?

    a. Vancomycin — Glycopeptide (cell wall)
    b. Ciprofloxacin — Quinolone (inhibit DNA synthesis)
    c. Penicillin G — penicillin (cell wall)
    d. Clindamycin — Macrolides (50s)
    e. Imipenem

3. Which antibiotic works by inhibiting peptidoglycan synthesis?

    a. Rifampacin
    b. Penicillin G
    c. Trimethoprim
    d. Ciproflozacin
    e. Tetracyclin

4. **What is the mechanism of action of low molecular weight heparin?**

   a. Inhibition of the carboxylation of factors II, VII, IX, X
   b. Factor Xa inhibitor
   c. Factor Xa activator
   d. Activation of antithrombin III
   e. Inhibition of antithrombin III

5. **Which of the following is INCORRECT about the use of Rivaroxaban?**

   a. Its mode of action is via factor Xa inhibition
   b. It is only available in oral form
   c. It is reported to be significantly more effective at preventing venous thromboembolism after total joint replacement than enoxaparin
   d. It is mainly renally excreted
   e. Protamine is an effective antidote

6. **What is the mode of action of the bisphosphonate drugs?**

   a. Macrophage inhibitor
   b. Osteoclast activator
   c. Osteoblast activator
   d. Osteoclast inhibitor
   e. Osteocyte inhibitors

7. **Which one of the following statements about calcitonin is INCORRECT?**

   a. Calcitonin is produced by the thyroid gland
   b. Calcitonin acts via osteoclasts
   c. Calcitonin can be used for treatment of Paget's disease and osteoporosis
   d. Calcitonin improves mineralisation of lytic lesions in myeloma
   e. Calcitonin lowers both calcium and phosphate serum levels

8. **Which one of the following statements is INCORRECT about parathyroid hormone (PTH)?**
   a. PTH acts to increase bone resorption
   b. Endogenous PTH is already in its active form at the point of secretion by the parathyroid gland
   c. Pulsed PTH is needed for bone formation
   d. PTH aids the production of activated Vitamin D
   5. PTH infusions are useful in patients with Paget's disease

9. **Which one of the following statements about the action of drugs is CORRECT?**
   a. Glucocorticoid action is mediated by a cAMP mechanism
   b. Aspirin is an irreversible inhibitor of COX
   c. COX 2 is a constituent form of the enzyme
   d. COX 2 inhibitors are associated with a reduced risk of cardio-vascular events
   e. Ibuprofen is an irreversible inhibitor of COX

10. **Which of the following statements are FALSE about rheuma-toid arthritis (RA)?**
    a. Cervical spine involvement is found in up to 80% of patients with RA
    b. Genetic linkage with HLA DR4 has been demonstrated
    c. Rheumatoid factor is an antibody directed against the Fc portion of IgG
    d. The viscosity of the fluid in the joints is increased compared to normal
    e. A characteristic feature of RA is the presence of TH1 cells in the synovium

11. **Which of the following is NOT associated with seronegative arthritis?**
    a. Chlamidia infection
    b. HLA B27
    c. Crohn's disease
    d. Psoriasis
    e. Necrobiosis lipoidica

12. **Which of the following is NOT true about calcium pyrophosphate dihydrate disease (pseudogout)?**
    a. It is strongly associated with hypercalcaemia
    b. The crystals are rhomboid shaped
    c. The crystals are negatively birefringent
    d. The wrist is commonly affected
    e. It may lead to secondary osteoarthritis

13. **Which of the following is NOT true about gout?**
    a. The serum uric acid level may be normal during an attack
    b. The crystals are strongly negatively birefringent rhomboid shaped crystals
    c. The first metatarsophalangeal joint is commonly affected
    d. Thiazide diuretics can precipitate an attack
    e. Allopurinol has no role in the treatment of an acute attack

14. **Which of the following is TRUE about Mycobacterium tuberculosis?**
    a. It stains deep purple in gram stain
    b. It can grow in anaerobic conditions
    c. The incidence is decreasing in the western world
    d. Rifampacin is second line treatment
    e. Rifampacin is a hepatic cytochrome P_{450} enzyme inducer

15. **What is the commonest organism found in an infection after a cat bite?**
    a. Group A Streptococcus
    b. Staphylococcus epidermidis
    c. Eikenella
    d. Pasteurella multocida
    e. Streptococcus pneumoniae

16. **Adalimumab and Infleximab are monoclonal antibodies that are used in the treatment of both seropositive and seronegative arthritis. Which answer best reflects their mode of action?**
    a. Monoclonal antibody designed to bind to TNF alpha
    b. Monoclonal antibody designed to bind to TNF alpha receptor
    c. Monoclonal antibody designed to bind to IL 1
    d. Monoclonal antibody designed to bind to IL 1 receptor
    e. Monoclonal antibody designed to bind to IL 6

17. **Which one of the following is the single most sensitive investigation in the diagnosis of total joint arthroplasty infection?**
    a. Bone scintography
    b. Radiolabelled white cell scan
    c. Serum CRP and white cell count
    d. Serum IL6 and activated protein C levels
    e. MRI Scan

18. **Which one of the following is a requirement for the establishment of a biofilm surrounding a total joint arthroplasty prosthesis?**
    a. Production of glycocalyx from planktonic bacteria
    b. Staphlycoccus aureus infection for at least six weeks
    c. Development of osteolytic lesions and the formation of a local acidic biological environment
    d. Exposed metalwork infected with mixed *Staph.* species
    e. Formation of extracellular polysaccharides including glycocalyces by organised bacterial colonies

19. **In an established prosthetic biofilm infection all of the following statements are true EXCEPT:**
    a. Organised colonies of bacteria are protected by an extracellular polysaccharide matrix including glycocalyx
    b. The formation of balloon colonies may seed the infection back into the joint following a period of quiescence
    c. Biofilms may form on bone as well as prosthesis surfaces
    d. Bacteria within the micro-environment of a biofilm are relatively protected from antibiotic action
    e. The biofilm may form in subclinical infection

20. **Which one of the following statements concerning infection in trauma is FALSE?**
    a. The infection rate in Gustillo-Anderson Grade 3C tibial fractures may reach 15% even with gold standard surgical management
    b. Insertion of a bone cement spacer following bone infection is associated with a lower subsequent infection rate
    c. Stainless steel implants are associated with a lower infection rate than titanium equivalents
    d. Maintenance of stability whilst suppressing infection is the primary goal in unhealed infected fractures
    e. Pin site infections may be associated with osteomyelitis in circular frame management of fractures

21. **A 23-year-old male presenting with sequestrum and a discharging sinus following a Gustillo-Anderson 3C open fracture of the femur is classified by the Cierny classification as:**
    a. Cierny class IIIB
    b. Cierny class IVA
    c. Cierny class IVB
    d. Cierny class IIA
    e. Cierny class IVA

22. **Which of the following treatment strategies has NOT been shown to decrease infection rate following open fractures?**
    a. Prompt administration of IV broad spectrum antibiotics
    b. Thorough wound debridement within 6 hours of injury
    c. Use of a 'cement bead pouch'
    d. Immediate restoration of blood supply
    e. Splintage and covering of the fracture

23. **Which of the following immunological responses is thought to mediate the development of aseptic lymphocytic vasculitis associated lesions (ALVAL)?**
    a. Type I hypersensitivity
    b. Type II hypersensitivity
    c. Type III hypersensitivity
    d. Type IV hypersensitivity
    e. Giant cell mediated response

24. **Which of the following has/have been shown to reduce rein-fection rates following revision hip surgery for prosthesis infection?**

    a. Two stage revision with the use of an antibiotic loaded spacer
    b. Extended post-operative i.v. antibiotic regimes
    c. Thorough local debridement of all infected tissue
    d. All of the above
    e. None of the above

25. **The final common pathway in osteolysis is:**

    a. Mediated by RANK receptors on the osteoclast surface membrane
    b. Caused by binding of OPG to a cell surface receptor on the osteoclast
    c. Mediated by IL-6 binding to osteoblasts
    d. Caused by RANK-L binding to OPG receptor on the osteoclast
    e. Not known

26. **Which of the following is associated with the initiation of the 'inflammatory' phase of fracture healing?**

    a. BMP 4
    b. FGF
    c. IL-6
    d. BMP 7
    e. TIMP 1 and 2

27. **Tuberculosis infection is associated with all of the following EXCEPT:**

    a. Caseating necrosis
    b. Giant dendritic cell formation
    c. Spinal collapse
    d. Cold abscess formation
    e. Indolent hip infection and femoral head collapse

28. **Which of the following organisms is/are most commonly associated with necrotising fasciitis?**
    a. E. coli with secondary Staphylococcus epidermis overgrowth
    b. Pseudomonas aeruginosa
    c. Clostridium difficile
    d. Streptococcus with Staphylococcus overgrowth
    e. Staphylococcus epidermidis

29. **Which one of the following is NOT a recognised clinical feature of necrotising fasciitis?**
    a. Localised pain and swelling
    b. Bullae and ischaemic skin changes
    c. Lymphangitis
    d. Signs of systemic sepsis
    e. Aggressive spreading cellulitis sometimes associated with surgical emphysema

Extended Matching Questions

SCENARIO I OPTIONS

A 1%

B 5%

C 15%

D 30%

E 50%

F 90%

G 100%

This question concerns fractures of the tibia. For each of the following questions choose the correct answer from the list above. Each answer may be used once, more than once or not at all.

1. What proportion of open tibial fractures requires input from a plastic surgeon during initial debridement?

2. What proportion of open tibial fractures will develop compartment syndrome in the peri-operative period?

3. What is the infection rate in surgically managed contaminated Gustilo-Anderson 3C open tibial fractures?

SCENARIO II OPTIONS

A Serum C-reactive protein and white cell count

B Bone scan and radiolabelled white cell scan

C Aspiration of the hip

D Single stage THR with extended antibiotic therapy

E Excision arthroplasty

F Two stage revision arthroplasty

G MRI Scan

Above is a list of investigations and interventions that may be undertaken in the assessment and management of a suspected hip infection. For each of the following scenarios select the single most appropriate next step from the list. Each answer may be used once, more than once or not at all.

4. A 73-year-old male of Indian origin has a confirmed diagnosis of tuberculosis of the hip. He has been treated with 3 months of triple therapy but then presents to the orthopaedic department with femoral head collapse.

5. A 4-year-old boy presents with a 4-hour history of limp, pyrexia and a painful tender hip. He is able to weight bear with difficulty.

6. A 72-year-old man presents with aggressive osteolytic change and a painful left total hip replacement. His CRP is 16 and WCC 11.

Answers: Chapter 6

MCQ 29
EMQ 6

Multiple Choice Answers

(handwritten: (Bacteraemias/enterobacter))

1. C Mechanism of action: *(handwritten: for aerobic gram -ve)*

Aminoglycosides: Inhibit the translocation of peptidyl-tRNA by binding to the 30S or 50S of the ribosome *(handwritten: Gent | Amikacin . renal excretn)*

Cephalosporins, glycopeptides, penicillins: Inhibit peptidoglycan cell wall synthesis *(handwritten: Cefuroxime 2 | ceftriaxone 3 G+/- Vancomycin — glycopeptide)*

Macrolides: Bind the 50S subunit of the ribosome to inhibit protein synthesis *(handwritten: G+ eg. Clarithromycin | erythromycin | azithromycin c. diff cause)*

(handwritten: Tendon rupture QT c.diff) **Quinolones:** inhibit DNA synthesis by acting on bacterial DNA gyrase. *(handwritten: Ciprofloxacin | levofloxacin G(+)/-)*

Sulphonamides: Inhibit folate synthesis

Tetracyclines: Bind to the 30S ribosomal subunit. They inhibit the binding of t-RNA to the ribosome. *(handwritten: broad spectrum doxycycline | tetracycline)*

Berg J., Tymoczko J., Stryer L. Biochemistry (Freeman 2011)

2. B The US FDA has administered warnings about the risk of Achillies' tendon rupture associated with the fluorquinolones. In addition fluoroquinolones are not licensed by the US FDA for use in children (except for treatment of anthrax!) due to the risk of mortality as well as permanent injury to the tendon/spontaneous tendon rupture. Whilst the evidence surrounding ciprofloxacin use and tendon rupture is poor (retrospective case series) there are supporting animal model studies.

3. B See question 1 for explanation.

4. B LMWH acts by inhibiting factor Xa. Its action cannot be measured by using the prothrombin time (extrinsic pathway; commonly used to monitor warfarin) or APTT (intrinsic pathway – affected by unfractionated heparin) but can be measured by anti-factor Xa activity. It cannot easily be reversed. The advantages over unfractionated heparin are that of a once-a-day dosing regimen and lower rates of heparin induced thrombocytopaenia (HIT).

By contrast unfractionated heparin acts via binding to and activating Antithrombin III. Antithrombin III is a major inhibitor of coagulation.

Warfarin inhibits the carboxylation of factors II, VII, IX, X.

5. E Rivaroxaban is the first direct oral factor Xa inhibitor. It was trialled in RECORD 1–4 in total joint replacement and has been reported to be more effective at reducing the rate of VTE than LMWH. It has been recommended by NICE for use in extended duration prophylaxis in total joint arthroplasty. Protamine can be used to neutralise the effects of heparin but not rivaroxaban, for which there is no antidote. The majority of clearance is via the kidneys.

6. D Bisphosphonates act on osteoclasts. The bisphosphonate binds to hydroxyapatite in the bone and then is ingested by the osteoclasts during remodelling. There are two modes of action, either the bisphosphonate inhibits the formation of the ruffled border; or there is direct induction of apoptosis in the osteoclast.

7. D Calcitonin is a hormone produced by the parafollicular cells (C-cells) of the thyroid. It is a polypeptide that is secreted in response to high serum calcium, pentagastrin and gastrin. Calcitonin acts directly on osteoclasts to reduce bone resorption and also inhibits calcium reabsorption from the gut and kidney.

Salmon calcitonin is used to treat post-menopausal osteoporosis, hypercalcaemia and Paget's disease. While calcitonin can improve pain in acute osteoporotic related vertebral fractures and in Paget's disease, a Cochrane review concluded that the evidence cannot support the use of calcitonin for the treatment of pain in bone metastases and does not improve mineralisation in myelomatous metastases.

Martinez-Zapata MJ, Roqué i Figuls M, Alonso-Coello P, Roman Y, Català E. Calcitonin for metastatic bone pain. Cochrane Database of Systematic Reviews 2006, Issue 3. Art. No.: CD003223. DOI: 10.1002/14651858.CD003223.pub2.

8. E Parathyroid hormone is a polypeptide hormone that is produced by the chief cells of the parathyroid glands. Its production is stimulated via low serum calcium and high serum phosphate. It acts on osteoblasts which in turn activate osteoclasts via RANK-L to enhance bone resorption. It also acts on the kidney to increase calcium reabsorption, produce activated vitamin D and increase phosphate losses. Continuously high levels can lead to osteoporosis, but pulsed exogenous PTH can be used to treat osteoporosis. It is contraindicated in the presence of Paget's disease due to the risk of osteosarcoma.

9. B Glucocorticoids are steroid hormones that target the nucleus of a cell, rather than working via a G protein mechanism.

All NSAIDs are reversible inhibitors of the COX enzyme, except aspirin which is an irreversible inhibitor. COX 2 inhibitors have an associated increased risk of cardiovascular side effects.

10. D Rheumatoid arthritis is an autoimmune systemic disease characterised by increased TH1 cell activity. There is a genetic linkage with HLA DR 4. Women are three times as commonly affected as men. C-spine involvement is as high as 80% but may be silent. The joint fluid viscosity is decreased compared with normal subjects. Rheumatoid factor is an antibody directed against the Fc portion of IgG and is present in 80% of cases.

11. E The seronegative arthritides are not associated with rheumatoid factor. They are classically Reiter's (associated with Chlamidial and GI infections), ankylosing spondylitis (HLA B27 associated), joint disease associated with psoriasis and arthritis associated with enteropathic disease (ulcerative colitis and Crohn's disease).

Necrobiosis lipoidica is a necrotising skin condition that usually occurs in patients with diabetes but may also be associated with rheumatoid arthritis.

12. C Calcium pyrophosphate dihydrate disease (pseudogout) is a polyarticular arthritis that commonly affects the wrist and knee joints. It is caused by the deposition of calcium pyrophosphate dehydrate in the joints. These crystals are weakly positively birefingent and rhomboid shaped. It is associated with hypercalcaemia and hypomagnesaemia.

13. B Gout is caused by the pathological deposition of uric acid crystals in tissues. The serum urate may not be elevated during an attack. The strongly negatively birefringent crystals are needle shaped, as opposed to the weakly positively birefringent rhomboid shaped crystals in pseudogout. In gout the first MTPJ is commonly affected. Thiazide and other diuretics, diet and physiological stress can precipitate an attack. Allopurinol is a treatment for chronic and not acute gout; it acts as a xanthine oxidase inhibitor.

14. C M. tuberculosis is a rod-shaped aerobic bacterium. It does not stain with gram stain as the cell wall prevents the stain from entering the cell, therefore staining with Ziehl-Neelsen is needed (an acid fast stain). The incidence is increasing in the Western world with the emergence of multidrug resistant strains. The first line treatment is with rifampacin, isoniazid, pyrazinamide and ethambutol. Rifampacin is a hepatic cytochrome P_{450} enzyme inducer which can affect other drugs, e.g. warfarin.

15. D The commonest bacteria isolated in infected wounds from human bites are Group A Streptococci. Eikenella is a commensal in the mouth and implicated in 'fight bite' infections. Pasteurella is implicated in cat and dog bites.

16. A Adalimumab and Infliximab are both monoclonal antibodies which target TNF alpha. They have been approved for use in the treatment of rheumatoid arthritis, psoriatic arthritis, enteropathic arthritis and ankylosing spondylitis. They are also used in the treatment of Crohn's disease.

17. C The most sensitive (but not specific) investigation for infection in total joint arthroplasty is the combination of serum markers of inflammation (CRP and WCC), showing over 98% sensitivity. The highest specificity is achieved by a combination of bone scintography and radiolabelled white cell scan.

18. E Planktonic bacteria freely float in suspension and do not form biofilms. A biofilm may form as rapidly as 24 hours. Osteolytic lesions are caused by infection, but not required for biofilm formation. Many bacterial species can form biofilms, and exposed metalwork is not specifically required.

19. **B** Breakaway colonies from biofilms are called 'streamers' not 'balloons'. Statements A, C, D and E are all true.

20. **C** Titanium debris has been demonstrated to be cytotoxic to bacteria and titanium implants have been shown to require a higher bacterial inoculation to result in established infection. All of the other statements are true.

21. **A** This is class III (sequestrum) with some local host compromise (type B) due to the vascular injury.

Cierny Classification

Type I: Medullary osteomyelitis with endosteal sinus

Type II: Superficial osteomyelitis

Type III: Well marginated sequestrum

Type IV: Permiative lesion often associated with instability

Host types

A – normal immune status

B – local compromise

C – significant immunocompromise.

22. **B** Although there have been a number of basic science studies looking at bacterial doubling times and contaminated wounds in animal models, there is no evidence for the 'six hour rule'; hence this is no longer included in the BOA/BAPRAS guidelines for management of open tibial fractures, whilst A, C, D and E are recommended.

23. **D** A range of immunological responses have been postulated as potential mechanisms in ALVAL formation following metal-on-metal hip arthroplasty. However, the presence of T-lymphocytes, as well as the expression of Type IV associated cytokines, has led to widespread acceptance of Type IV hypersensitivity as by far the most likely mechanism.

24. **D** Although some centres are now advocating single stage revision without the use of extended prophylaxis or antibiotic loaded spacers, the highest cure rates have been shown to be associated with 2-stage revision, undertaking thorough debridement and using antibiotic loaded spacers in combination with extended i.v. antibiotic administration.

25. **A** The RANK-RANK-L receptor sits on the osteoclast and mediates the loss of bone associated with osteolysis. OPG is the soluble inhibitor for this receptor.

26. **B** FGF-2 is associated with the initial inflammatory of bone healing. IL-6 is a B-cell mediator and plays no part in fracture healing. The BMPs and their inhibitors (TIMPs – tissue inhibitors of metallopro-teinases) are expressed later in the fracture healing process. BMP-4 plays no role in fracture healing, and the other BMPs play a greater role in the later stages of fracture healing.

27. **B** The histological findings in tuberculosis include dentritic cells and giant cells which both form from macrophage pre-cursor cells.

28. **D** There are four recognised types of necrotising fasciitis. The commonest is a Group A Streptococcus with anaerobic overgrowth.

The types of necrotising fasciitis are:

Type 1: Polymycrobial infection with aerobic and anaerobic

Type 2: Group A Streptococcus with staphylococcus overgrowth

Type 3: Gram negative polymicrobial infection

Type 4: Fungal infection

29. **C** Necrotising fasciitis is invariably a very aggressive clinical entity, and as such is therefore almost never associated with lymphangitis.

Extending Matching Answers

1. G The new BOA/BAPRAS guidelines emphasise the importance of dual assessment for all open tibial fractures during the initial assessment phase.

2. B It is a widely held misconception that compartment syndrome cannot occur in the presence of an open fracture. However, between 2 and 6% of open tibial fractures are known to develop compartment syndrome.

3. C Figures vary in different series, but even with gold standard management the infection rate in open tibial fractures with associated vascular injury approaches 15%. The lowest reported rates in the literature are 5%, with the highest 30%.

4. D Tuberculous infection of the hip can be successfully treated with primary THR with subsequent extended antimicrobial therapy.

5. A There is no indication to move directly to hip aspiration without first checking this patient's inflammatory markers. If a patient has three out of pyrexia, inability to weight bear, raised inflammatory markers and elevated white cell count there is a greater than 90% likelihood of septic arthritis.

6. C This patient is likely to have an infected hip prosthesis. However, in the presence of borderline blood tests the diagnosis can be confirmed by aspiration. Identification of the organism prior to revision surgery in cases of suspected infection also allows accurate planning of subsequent antibiotic prophylaxis.

Chapter 7

Ligaments and Tendons

> MCQ 24
> EMQ 6

Multiple Choice Questions

1. The ligamentum flavum is a specialised ligament which has a high elastin content. The effect of this high elastin content is to:

   a. Increase the toe effect due to the increased elastin content, and provide the tension-band effect to the spine

   b. Increase the ultimate tensile strength and breaking point of the ligament

   c. Form increased hydrogen bonds between the collagen fibres, thereby increasing the toughness of the ligament

   d. Create a large zone where Hooke's law is followed, with reduced elastic recoil to prevent crumpling into the spinal canal

   e. Increase the hysteresis effect due to increased heat loss during loading

2. **The differences in biomechanical properties of immature tendon and bone are responsible for the relatively high preponderance of avulsion fractures in the paediatric population as compared with adults. Which one of the following best explains this phenomenon?**
   a. Immature bone has increased viscoelastic properties; at high strain rates the Young's modulus increases resulting in a higher strength and ultimate tensile strength than ligament
   b. Immature ligament has increased viscoelastic properties; at high strain rates the Young's modulus increases resulting in a higher strength and ultimate tensile strength than bone
   c. Immature ligament has increased collagen content and a larger toe region; this results in a weaker ligament which fails with an avulsion fracture
   d. Immature ligament has increased collagen content and a larger toe region; this results in a stronger ligament causing the bone to fail preferentially
   e. Immature ligament has increased elastin content and a larger toe region; this results in a stronger ligament causing the bone to fail preferentially

3. **Concerning the viscoelastic properties of ligament, which of the following statements is FALSE?**
   a. Viscous properties predominate at low strain rates
   b. Elastic properties are seen at high strain rates
   c. Stress relaxation occurs when constant stress is applied for a prolonged period of time
   d. The load-elongation curve differs in loading and unloading
   e. There is an increased strain in response to a constant application of stress

4. **With regards to injuries to ligaments and tendons, which of the following statements is/are FALSE?**

   a. Ligaments and tendons share a common injury grading system
   b. Grade I tears (mild) occur following micro trauma and failure of collagen fibrils. However there is no joint laxity
   c. Grade II injuries (moderate) progressive failure of collagen fibrils and partial rupture has occurred. Some laxity is detectable
   d. Grade III injuries (severe) display no resistance to stress on examination
   e. All of the above are incorrect statements

5. **Which one of the following factors is NOT recognised as modulating the biomechanical properties of ligaments?**

   a. Increasing age
   b. Endocrine changes
   c. Pharmacological factors
   d. Eccentric loading
   e. Mobilisation

6. **All of the following statements concerning the effects of aging on ligaments are true EXCEPT:**

   a. During maturation the number and quality of hydrogen bond cross-links increase resulting in increased tensile strength
   b. After maturation the mean collagen diameter and content decrease resulting in a decline in mechanical properties
   c. Mid-substance failure tends to occur in an adult ligament due to the stress concentration at the weakest point
   d. Sharpey's fibres are located in the zone of transition between ligament and bone at the mineralised fibrocartilage layer. These are stronger in children resulting in avulsion fractures
   e. During life there is a gradual decline in the biomechanical strength of ligaments resulting in a higher rate of injury in older men and women

7. **Which of the following statements concerning Achilles' tendinopathy is TRUE?**

   a. Repetitive micro-trauma results in micro-tears and an inflammatory response, which in turn lead to localised calcification. The consequent alteration in biomechanical properties can result in rupture

   b. Overload of the tendon results in injury to the paratenon and subsequent circumferential inflammation. This results in an increased fluid content in the tendon, which may lead to subsequent rupture

   c. Aging of the Achilles' tendon results in increased fluid content, increased stiffness and a subsequent inflammatory response, but no increased risk of rupture

   d. Hypercalcaemia results in calcification of the tendon, inducing a localised inflammatory response in the paratenon

   e. Higher load rates associated with stiffer older tissue can result in microtrauma and subsequent trauma and microfracture

8. **Which of the following most accurately reflects the dry weight of tendon?**

   a. 25% collagen which is synthesised by tenocytes to form longitudinal and transverse fibres

   b. 50% collagen which is synthesised by tenocytes to form longitudinal and transverse fibres

   c. 75% collagen which is synthesised by tenocytes to form longitudinal and transverse fibres

   d. 50% collagen which is synthesised by fibrocytes to form a longitudinal quartile staggered array

   e. 25% collagen which is synthesised by fibrocytes to form a longitudinal quartile staggered array

9. **With regards to tendon healing which of the following statements is FALSE?**

   a. During the inflammatory phase initial healing begins with haematoma formation
   b. Clot formation releases inflammatory mediators and chemotactic factors
   c. During the proliferative phase macrophage and fibroblast infiltration and replication begin with formation of new extracellular matrix
   d. Fibroblasts continue rapid proliferation and synthesis of collagens, proteoglycans, and type III collagen
   e. During the remodelling phase there is a decrease in cellularity, reduced matrix synthesis, decrease in type III collagen, and an increase in type I collagen synthesis

10. **With regards to growth factors implicated in repair of tendons which of the following has NOT been implicated in tendon healing?**

    a. IGF-1
    b. TGF Beta
    c. PDGF
    d. VEGF
    e. IL-6

11. **Which one of the following types of collagen types is the predominant type of collagen type in ligaments?**

    a. I
    b. II
    c. III
    d. VI
    e. X

12. **Which one of the following is a difference between ligaments and tendons?**
    a. Only tendons have a toe region on their stress strain curve
    b. Only ligaments exhibit stress-relaxation properties
    c. Tendons have a more ordered collagen structure
    d. Ligaments have a lower ground substance content
    e. Tendons have a lower collagen content

13. **Which one of the following responses is TRUE about ligament attachments to bones?**
    a. Ligaments insert into bone more commonly via direct than indirect insertions
    b. An indirect insertion consists of collagen, fibrocartilage, mineralised fibrocartilage, bone
    c. In a direct insertion the ligament is anchored to bone via Sharpey's fibres
    d. Ligaments are avascular at their attachments
    e. At low rates of strain, ligaments tend to fail at insertion in the mature skeleton

14. **Which one of the following is TRUE about tendons?**
    a. Elastin concentration in tendon on average is greater than that of ligaments
    b. Tendon substance contains many cells
    c. Young's modulus irrevocably decreases with age
    d. Midsubstance tears are more common than myotendinous unit or avulsion ruptures
    e. Tendons have a good nerve supply

15. **Which one of the following is CORRECT about the ultrastructure of tendons?**
    a. Collagen fibres are arranged in an oblique manner for strength
    b. The secondary structure is right handed
    c. The tertiary structure is left handed
    d. The quaternary structure is quartile staggered
    e. Collagen I is composed of four chains in helical array

16. **Which one of the following is CORRECT about the stress-strain curve of tendons?**
    a. After the initial toe region, with increasing stress the stress-strain curve flattens
    b. The toe region is part of the plastic deformation of the tendon
    c. The presence of elastin is responsible for the toe region
    d. The plastic region has spikes due to sequential fibre rupture
    e. Elastic modulus increases with age

17. **Which one of the following statements about ACL reconstruction is CORRECT?**
    a. Bone-patella-bone graft healing to tunnels is complete by 12 weeks
    b. Bone-patella-bone graft healing occurs with Sharpey's fibres
    c. Hamstring tendon grafts heal by direct insertion into bone tunnels
    d. Hamstring tendon grafts heal by indirect insertion into bone tunnels
    e. All of the above

18. **Which one of the following is INCORRECT about the healing of an immobilised ligament?**
    a. The predominant collagen in the healed tendon is type I
    b. Remodelling increases type I collagen
    c. Type III collagen is stronger due to its random organisation than type I
    d. Healing ligament is hypocellular and disorganised
    e. In the adjacent normal ligament the structural properties fall with inactivity

19. **Which one of the following is CORRECT about the effect of immobilisation upon the properties of ligaments?**
    a. Immobilisation results in increased stiffness
    b. Immobilisation results in increased strength
    c. Immobilisation results in increased stiffness and no effect on strength
    d. Immobilisation has no effect upon the mechanical properties
    e. Immobilsation results in decreased stiffness and strength

20. Which of one the following is NOT a histological feature of tendinosis?

a. Collagen degeneration
b. Hypercellularity
c. Vascular ingrowth
d. Absence of inflammatory cells
e. Decreased interfibrillary glycosaminoglycan concentration

21. Which one of the following is NOT true about the healing of tendons?

a. Collagen synthesis is detected at the earliest at 14 days
b. At 3-4 weeks the remodelling begins
c. Paratenon-covered tendons heal more reliably than sheathed tendons
d. There are three phases of tendon healing
e. At 20 weeks the tendon histologically resembles normal tendon

22. Which of the following is TRUE about the effect of an anterior opening wedge high tibial osteotomy on the knee?

a. The resting position of the tibia is moved posteriorly with respect to the femur
b. The resting position of the tibia is unchanged
c. The stress on the ACL increases
d. The stress on the PCL increases
e. There is no change in the stress on the ACL or PCL

23. Which of the following is TRUE about the healing of flexor tendons in the hand?

a. The flexor tendons are covered by a paratenon
b. The paratenon produces synovial fluid
c. The blood supply comes from the paratenon
d. Areas of relative avascularity within the tendon compromise healing
e. Early primary tendon repair gives poorer results than secondary reconstruction

24. Following a painful non-contact twisting injury to the knee a patient is assessed in clinic. The patient is relaxed and a good examination is possible. The examiner finds that there is increased laxity on the Lachman test but a normal pivot shift. The PCL is intact, as are all other structures within the knee. Which bundle(s) of the ACL have/has been damaged?

    a. Neither anteromedial and posterolateral torn
    b. Anteromedial tear with intact posterolateral
    c. Posterolateral tear with intact anteromedial
    d. Anterolateral tear with intact posteromedial
    e. Anterolateral intact with posteromedial tear

Extended Matching Questions

SCENARIO I OPTIONS

A Type I collagen

B Type II collagen

C Type III collagen

D Type IV collagen

E Type V collagen

F Type IV collagen

G Type X collagen

From the options above, correctly choose the type of collagen found in each of the following scenarios. Each answer may be used once, more than once or not at all.

1. The major fibrillar component of tendon.

2. Forms cross-links to other collagen types and regulates the characteristics of fibrillar structures in tendon.

3 The major component of endotenon and epitenon.

SCENARIO II OPTIONS

A Musculotendinous junction
B Osseotendinous junction
C Extracellular matrix
D Proteoglycans
E Elastin

F Fibroblasts
G Tenocytes
H Collagenocytes
I Histiocytes

Above is a list of micro- and macroscopic structures and sites within the adult mature tendon. For each of the following description choose the correct site. Each answer may be used once, more than once or not at all.

4. Contains a dense collection of collagen fibres and tenocytes within a well ordered matrix.

5. The predominant cell type in the tendon; responsible for synthesis and maintenance of the extracellular matrix.

6. An integral part of the extracellular matrix that functions to stabilise the collagen fibres.

Answers: Chapter 7

MCQ 24
EMQ 6

Multiple Choice Answers

1. D Hooke's law states that stress is proportional to strain; this is followed in the elastic zone of the stress-strain curve. The higher elastin content of the ligamentum flavum elongates this zone but does not dramatically affect its other biomechanical properties. It has the secondary effect of preventing buckling into the canal. The tension band principle is maintained by the posterior muscles attached to the spinous processes.

2. B Strength is the area under the stress-strain curve. The increased viscoelastic properties of immature ligament mean that a greater stress is required for the ligament to ruture than the bone to fracture. Young's modulus, E, is a material property describing its 'stiffness' (although for the purist they are not the same thing), and is given by the gradient of the stress-strain curve in the elastic region.

3. C Viscoelastic materials demonstrate both rate-dependent and time-dependent properties. Stress relaxation occurs when ligament (or other viscoelastic material) is exposed to constant strain (defined as change in length over original length) for a prolonged period of time, and is defined as a time-dependent decrease in the stress in the material for a constantly applied strain.

4. E Statements A–D are correct; the grading system commonly used is as described. E is therefore incorrect.

Grade 1	Occurs following micro-trauma and failure of collagen fibrils. No joint laxity
Grade 2	Progressive failure of collagen fibrils with accompanying partial rupture. Some detectable laxity
Grade 3	Complete rupture

5. D Eccentric loading is a type of exercise where muscle lengthening occurs whilst still under load. Although associated with tendon injury, it is not a recognised mechanism for alteration of biomechanical properties. Conversely, the biomechanical properties of ligaments and tendons have been demonstrated to be significantly reduced with increasing age, and also with the administration of local steroid injections. Systemic non-steroidals have also been shown to affect the tensile strength of ligaments, although there remains some debate as to whether the net result is an increase or decrease. Fluctuations in female endocrine profile during pregnancy, as well as the different stages of the menstrual cycle, are known to increase ligamentous laxity, and mobilisation following tendon injury has a role in the promotion of remodelling, with an associated increase in tensile strength.

6. D Sharpey's fibres form part of the insertion of ligaments into bone. However, they are not responsible for the rate of avulsion fractures in children; this is due to the relatively superior mechanical properties of paediatric ligament compared to bone.

7. A As stated, repeated micro-trauma leads to microscopic damage and a resultant inflammatory response, with associated calcification. The resulting alteration in biomechanical properties can result in rupture.

8. C Although 70% water *in vivo*, the solid component of tendon is predominantly collagen, which comprises 75% of the dry weight (mainly type I). Tenocytes have a primarily synthetic function, and although the collagen is mostly organised into longitudinal spiral fibres in a quartile-staggered array there are also transverse collagen fibrils found in tendon. The remainder of the solid component comprises elastin, ground substances and collagen types III and IV.

9. C

Macrophage infiltration and formation of new matrix occur during the inflammatory phase. The distinct phases of tendon healing may be summarised as follows:

Inflammatory: Initial healing begins with haematoma formation. Clot formation releases inflammatory mediators and chemotactic factors. Macrophage and fibroblast infiltration and replication begins with formation of new ECM.

Proliferative: Fibroblasts continue rapid proliferation and synthesis of collagens, proteoglycans, and type III collagen. There is a rapid increase in cellularity and collagen concentration.

Remodelling: A decrease in cellularity, reduced matrix synthesis, decrease in type III collagen, and an increase in type I collagen synthesis.

10. E IL-6 is a systemic T-cell mediated inflammatory cytokine, but has not been shown to play a role in the healing process following tendon injury.

11. A Type I collagen is the predominant collagen type in bone, tendon, and ligaments.

Type II collagen is the predominant type in hyaline cartilage.

Type III collagen is present in smaller amounts and is also present in early scar tissue, Dupuytren's disease and early callus.

Type VI is present in large concentrations in intervertebral discs and type X is present in mineralised cartilage and important in ossification.

12. C Ligaments and tendons are similar with some important differences:

Similarities
- They are both composed of type I collagen, proteoglycans and water
- Both exhibit a toe region to the stress strain curve as the crimped fibres elongate
- Both exhibit viscoelastic behaviour
- Both have the fibroblast as the predominant cell type

Differences
- The average ligament has a lower concentration of type I collagen (up to 70% of total collagen in ligaments and 95% of total collagen in tendons – dry weight), but a higher percentage of proteoglycans and water
- The collagen in tendon is more organised
- Tendon collagen fibres are less crimped therefore there is a smaller toe region on the stress strain curve

13. **A** Ligaments and tendons have a similar morphology in their insertion into bone. The direct insertion (more common in ligaments) has collagen fibres going through four stages of insertion (collagen fibres, fibrocartilage, calcified fibrocartilage and bone) e.g. cruciate ligaments. In indirect attachments Sharpey's fibres (collagen fibres that pass from the ligament/tendon via the periosteum) are present. An example is the tibial insertion of the superficial MCL of the knee. Indirect attachments are common in short ligaments or tendons that have broad attachments and are more common in tendons. The blood supply to ligaments is sparse and concentrated at the insertion points.

There are three failure mechanisms for ligaments which are determined by strain rate. The first is midsubstance tearing of the ligament, which tends to happen at high strain rates, the second occurs at lower strain rates when there tends to be a failure at the ligament – bone interface (novice skier getting off a chair lift, ACL torn from femoral insertion site), finally there are bony avulsion fractures, which again occur at low strain rates (or in the paediatric population).

14. **E** Tendons and ligaments have few cells, but both contain fibroblasts as the predominant cell type (also called tenocytes in tendons, although not strictly identical in every case), which are more numerous in tendons and are flatter in shape. The elastin concentration in tendon is approximately 2%, whereas in ligaments it can range from 5–47 %. Tendons tend to have higher pyridinoline content.

In a normal tendon, failure at either the bone or the musculotendinous junction is more common than midsubstance failure. The Young's modulus of tendons decreases with age but can be reversed with strength training. Tendons also have a rich nerve supply at their insertions that are typically innervated by the nerve to the associated muscle.

Reeves N et al. Effect of strength training on human patella tendon mechanical properties of older individuals May 1, 2003 The Journal of Physiology, 548, 971–981

15. D The primary structure of collagen is a characteristic tri-aminoacid sequence. Every third residue is glycine with the other residues frequently being proline or hydroxyproline. The secondary structure is a narrow left-handed helix (alpha chain). In the tertiary structure, three separate alpha chains (2 identical alpha 1 and one alpha 2 chain) form a right-handed rod-like superhelix. Finally the collagen arranges itself in a quartile staggered array.

16. D Under low stress the tendon is compliant and exhibits a toe region as the crimped fibres uncrimp. The tendons then have a near linear elastic region (where they display viscoelasticity). The curve in this region is steeper than the toe region. After the elastic region there is a plastic region where there is sequential failure of tendon fibres giving rise to spikes on the stress – strain curve before eventual failure. The elastic modulus of tendon decreases with age, an effect that can be reversed with resistive training.

17. E Bone-patella-bone grafts heal by two mechanisms; the first is bone to bone healing as per fracture healing; the second is via Sharpey's fibres linking the soft tissue portion of the graft to the tunnels. Hamstring grafts have been shown to heal by both direct and indirect insertions.

Weiler A. et al. Tendon healing in a bone tunnel. Part 1. Biomechanical results after biodegradable interference fit fixation in a model of anterior cruciate ligament reconstruction in sheep. Arthroscopy 2002;(18) 2:113–123

Malinin T. et al. A study of retrieved allografts used to replace anterior cruciate ligaments Arthroscopy 2002 18 (2) 163–170

18. D For ligaments and tendons there are three phases of healing:

1. **Inflammatory** – Immediately after injury a fibrin clot forms with inflammatory cells infiltrating the zone of injury with the release of inflammatory and chemotactic mediators.

2. **Proliferative** – Fibroblasts migrate into the defect and state to produce extracellular matrix and large amounts of type III collagen. This collagen is disorganised but highly cellular. The type III collagen is weak and the tendon is at its weakest point in the repair process.

3. **Remodelling** – Type III collagen is remodelled into type I collagen by the action of the matrix metalloproteinases. This phase can last months to years and may never result in complete restitution.

19. E Joint immobility results in an exponential decrease in the mechanical properties of ligaments in a matter of weeks. With the recommencement of exercise the mechanical properties improve back to pre-immobilisation levels but recovery takes far longer than the rate of deterioration. Conversely the loading of aging tendons can significantly improve the mechanical properties thereby demonstrating plasticity in myotendinous performance.

20. E Tendinosis is associated with various histological changes. These include absence of inflammatory cells, vascular ingrowth, collagen degeneration, disordered fibres, hypercellularity and increased interfibrillar glycosaminoglycans.

21. A Type III collagen synthesis can be detected as early as 3 days following injury. Gradually the gap between the tendons is filled with collagen fibres. At 3–4 weeks remodelling starts and is associated with improvements in the mechanical properties of the tendons. As the remodelling phase progresses the mechanical properties improve and histologically there is an increase in type I collagen, which is laid down in parallel with the lines of stress. At the same time there is a decrease in the cellularity and vascularity of the healing tissue. At 20 weeks the tendon histologically resembles normal tendon although the mechanical properties may never be normal.

Paratenon-covered tendons have a better blood supply and heal more reliably than sheathed tendons that have avascular segments, which rely upon diffusion for nutrients.

22. E An anterior opening wedge high tibial osteotomy increases the posterior tibial slope. This in turn moves the resting position of the tibia anteriorly with respect to the femur. There is no change in the stress in either ACL or PCL in either flexion or extension. However it improves stability in the chronically PCL deficient knee and can reconstitute the missing 'tibial step'.

Giffin R et al. Effects of Increasing Tibial Slope on the Biomechanics of the Knee Am J Sports Med 2004, 32 (2), 376–382

23. **D** The flexor tendons of the hand are covered by a synovial sheath that produces synovial fluid to reduce friction. They are not covered by a paratenon. The blood supply comes from the bony insertions and from vinculae running in the sheath. This means that there are relatively avascular areas within the tendon (zone 2 hand flexor tendons) and nutrition is gained by diffusion from the synovial fluid. Early primary repair gives better results than delayed repair.

24. **B** The ACL reportedly has two main bundles, the anteromedial and posterolateral. The anteromedial has been reported to control the anterior translation of the tibia on femur, as evaluated by the Lachman test, whereas the posterolateral bundle is probably more important in controlling rotatory instability, assessed in the pivot shift test. The posterolateral bundle has negligible effect on controlling anterior translation. An isolated injury to either bundle is possible but clinical examination based on the Lachman test alone is not able to distinguish between complete ACL rupture and an isolated anteromedial tear.

Christel P et al. The contribution of each anterior cruciate ligament bundle to the Lachman testa cadaver investigation J Bone Joint Surg Br January 2012 vol. 94–B no. 1, 68–74.

Extending Matching Answers

1. A

2. E

3. C

Collagen Type	Functional location
I	Bone, tendon, meniscus
II	Articular Cartilage
III	Epitenon/paratenon and early repair
IV	Basement membrane
V	Cross linkage
VIII	Epithelial cells
X	Mineralisation of cartilage

4. A The musculotendinous junction contains high numbers of tenocytes and fibroblasts.

5. F There are two cellular components to tendon – tenocytes and fibroblasts. Tenocytes are spindle-shaped fibroblast-like cells that are responsible for the synthesis of pre-collagen; this is assembled into the collagen fibrils in the extra-cellar matrix. Fibroblasts are situated between the fibrils in the extracellular matrix and synthesise and maintain the matrix.

6. E Although elastin has significant elastic properties, its function in tendon is to stabilise the collagen fibrils during stretch. Other glycopeptides such as aggrecan are responsible for maintaining water content and resisting repeated load cycles.

Chapter 8

Biomaterials and Tribology

MCQ 21
EMQ 13

Multiple Choice Questions

1. Which one of the following is NOT true about the mechanical properties of bone?
   a. Its stiffness increases with rate of strain
   b. It demonstrates anisotropic behaviour
   c. It demonstrates hysteretic behaviour
   d. It demonstrates creep
   e. Dehydration decreases the brittleness of bone

2. The cold working of stainless steel does NOT afford which one of the following properties?
   a. Increased hardness
   b. Increased toughness
   c. Decreased ductility
   d. Decreased Young's modulus
   e. Increased tensile strength

3. Which of the following changes does NOT occur with the cross linking of ultra-high molecular weight polyethylene (UHMWPE) with irradiation?
   a. Decreased wear rate
   b. Decreased Young's modulus
   c. Decreased ductility
   d. Decreased ultimate tensile strength
   e. Decreased fracture toughness

4. Which of the following terms does NOT describe the properties of synovial fluid?

   a. Non-Newtonian
   b. Pseudoplastic
   c. Shear thinning
   d. Thixotropic
   e. Rheopectic

5. Which of the following methods of lubrication is thought to occur in traditional artificial joints?

   a. Boundary lubrication
   b. Elastohydrodynamic lubrication
   c. Boosted lubrication
   d. Weeping lubrication
   e. Microelastohydrodynamic lubrication

6. Which of the following methods of lubrication is thought to occur in a well-functioning large diameter head metal-on-metal hip replacement during the swing phase?

   a. Boundary lubrication
   b. Elastohydrodynamic lubrication
   c. Hydrodynamic lubrication
   d. Weeping lubrication
   e. Microelastohydrodynamic lubrication

7. Regarding polyethylene wear in a well-functioning total hip replacement, which one of the following is the predominant type of wear?

   a. Fatigue
   b. Third body
   c. Adhesive wear
   d. Abrasive wear
   e. Backside wear

8. **For which one of the following materials is the gradient of its stress strain curve numerically similar to cancellous bone?**
   a. Polymethylmethacrylate (PMMA)
   b. Titanium
   c. Ceramic
   d. Stainless steel
   e. Cobalt chrome

9. **The advantages of a ceramic head over a metal head for a total hip replacement include:**
   a. Lower wettability
   b. Greater brittleness
   c. Greater malleability
   d. Longer plastic region on stress-strain curve
   e. Increased surface hardness

10. **The unwanted loss of metal ions into a solution via electron transfer between two electrochemically different metals in physical contact via the solution is called:**
    a. Galvanic corrosion
    b. Pitting corrosion
    c. Fretting corrosion
    d. Stress corrosion
    e. Crevice corrosion

11. **The distance between two screws positioned on either side of a fracture in a compression plate is known as:**
    a. Working length
    b. Pitch
    c. Core diameter
    d. Screw lead
    e. Area moment of inertia

12. **Which one of the following materials can undergo self-passivation?**

    a. Titanium
    b. Bone
    c. Polyethylene
    d. Ceramic
    e. Stainless steel

13. **Which of the following factors does NOT affect the pullout strength of cancellous bone screws?**

    a. Core and thread diameter
    b. Cannulation
    c. Screw thread depth
    d. Screw thread pitch
    e. Whether the screw is self-tapping or not

14. **Which one of the following is the best definition for 'the endurance limit'?**

    a. The stress at which a material can withstand an infinite number of cyclical loads without failure
    b. The stress at which permanent deformation of the material occurs
    c. The stress at which the material breaks
    d. The area under the stress strain curve up to the failure point
    e. The end of the linear region of the stress-strain curve

15. **Which one of the following properties is NOT a characteristic of a viscoelastic material?**

    a. Creep
    b. Strain rate dependency
    c. Stress relaxation
    d. Hysteresis
    e. Resistance to wear

16. **Which one of the following is the best definition of forging?**
    a. The pouring of a molten metal into a mould before letting it cool
    b. The use of force to drive solid metal into a mould to make it conform to the shape
    c. Heating the metal to a temperature below its melting point and then allowing it to cool at a predetermined rate
    d. Plastically deforming a metal to improve its material properties, usually at room temperature
    e. Forcing a material through a die to create a shape of desired cross section

17. **Which one of the following is NOT a constituent of PMMA bone cement?**
    a. A liquid methylmethacrylate monomer
    b. Hydroxyquinone acting to inhibit polymerisation
    c. N,N-dimethyl-p-toluidine acting as an accelerant
    d. Dibenzoyl peroxide acting as an inhibitor
    e. $BaSO_4$ / ZrO_2 acting as a radiopacifier

18. **Which one of the following materials can undergo phase transformation?**
    a. Titanium
    b. Alumina
    c. Zirconia
    d. Tantalum
    e. Stainless steel

19. **Which one of the following materials can undergo galvanic corrosion in the human body?**
    a. Cobalt chrome
    b. Pure titanium
    c. Pure alumina
    d. Tantalum
    e. Hydroxyapatite

20. **Which particle size produced by the wear of polyethylene is most biologically active in generating osteolysis in a total hip arthroplasty?**
    a. <0.1 μm
    b. $0.1–1$ μm
    c. $1–10$ μm
    d. $10–100$ μm
    e. >100 μm

21. **Which one of the following determines the bioactivity of polyethylene particles in osteolysis surrounding total joint replacements?**
    a. Particle size
    b. Particle number
    c. Particle shape
    d. Particle material
    e. All of the above

Extended Matching Questions

SCENARIO I OPTIONS

A Creep
B Viscoelasticity
C Stiffness
D Strain

E Stress
F Stress relaxation
G Strength

Which of the options above best fits the definition in each question? Each option may be used once, more than once or not at all.

1. Continued deformation under a constant or cyclical stress.

2. The resistance of a structure to deformation.

3. Normalized measure of deformation representing the displacement between particles in the body relative to a reference length.

4. Average force per unit area of a surface within the body on which forces act.

5. The ability of a material to withstand an applied stress without failure.

6. Reduction in stress in response to constant strain.

SCENARIO II OPTIONS

A Selenium   E Chromium
B Cobalt   F Vanadium
C Alumina   G Molybdenum
D Tantalum

Which of the options above best fits the definition in each question? Each option may be used once, more than once or not at all.

7. Which material demonstrates notch sensitivity?

8. Which material best demonstrates wettability?

9. Which principal material is added to steel to increase its resistance to corrosion?

10. Which material is added to steel to increase its hardness?

11. Which material is commonly added to titanium to increase its hardness?

12. Which material has greatest biocompatability and can be used in a porous form?

13. Which material is produced by hot isostatic pressing?

Answers: Chapter 8

MCQ 21
EMQ 13

Multiple Choice Answers

1. E Bone is viscoelastic, therefore its mechanical properties are dependent upon strain rate (rate of change in length), they are also dependent upon state of hydration and temperature. The viscoelastic features of bone are strain rate dependency, hysteresis and creep. Materials that have mechanical properties that are the same in all directions are isotropic, e.g. metals and ceramic. By contrast most biological tissue exhibits mechanical properties that are dependent upon the direction of applied stress, so called anisotropic behaviour.

Dehydration of bone increases its brittleness. All the other characteristics listed are viscoelastic properties of bone. Viscoelastic means that it exhibits viscous behaviour (time dependent, as discussed above) and elastic behaviour (returns to its original shape after the deforming force has been removed).

2. D Cold working of a material is the plastic deformation of a material carried out at a temperature below its melting point. The aim is to improve its strength.

When stainless steel is cold worked the microstructure alters with a reduction in grain size and increase in grain dislocations. The advantages are increased strength and surface hardness. Yield and ultimate stress are increased but the ductility is decreased. There is no change to the Young's modulus.

3. B One of methods of sterilising UHMWPE is by gamma irradiation. A side effect of radiation is free radical production, which is often combined with low melt annealing to result in crosslinkage of the polyethylene. The radiation breaks the carbon-hydrogen and carbon-carbon bonds and results in free radical generation resulting in either chain scission or the more advantageous cross linking. The effects of cross linking upon the properties of UHMWPE are increased Young's modulus, decreased ductility, decreased ultimate tensile strength, decreased fracture toughness and decreased wear rate.

4. E Synovial fluid is produced by type B synoviocytes. It exhibits non-Newtonian fluid behaviour.

A Newtonian fluid is one in which stress is proportional to the rate of strain. Synovial fluid has non-Newtonian behavior as it is thixotropic. This means that its viscosity (the gradient of the stress versus strain rate curve) decreases with duration of stress (a time dependent feature). Some other relevant terms are defined as follows:

- Shear thinning – viscosity decreases with increasing stress (time independent behaviour) (synonym – pseudoplastic)
- Shear thickening – viscosity increases with increasing stress (time independent behaviour) (synonym – dilatant)
- Rheopectic – viscosity increases with duration of stress (time dependent)

5. A Boundary lubrication: the applied load is carried by the articular surface with a very thin layer of fluid in between to reduce friction and wear. The lambda ratio is less than 1. The boundary molecule is lubricin which also has a role in reducing friction. This form of lubrication predominates in most hard-on-soft bearings.

(In reality a combination of fluid film and boundary lubrication coexists – so called mixed lubrication.)

Fluid-film lubrication: the applied load is fully supported by a fluid film in between the joint surfaces that prevents asperity contact. The ratio of fluid film thickness to roughness of a surface is measured as the lambda ratio. For fluid-film lubrication the lambda ratio has to be greater than 3. This type predominates in synovial joints.

Hydrodynamic lubrication is a type of fluid film lubrication where a wedge of fluid separates the surfaces. The speed of movement of the surface, the applied force and the viscosity of the fluid are all important factors. There is evidence that thick film or hydrodynamic lubrication occurs with hard-on-hard hip bearings with large heads and appropriate radial clearances.

Elastohydrodynamic lubrication is a type of fluid film lubrication in which elastic deformation of the bearing surface (e.g cartilage) occurs dissipating the applied load over a greater fluid film area. In micro-elastohydrodynamic lubrication the asperities of articular cartilage are smoothed improving the lambda ratio.

Squeeze film lubrication occurs when a fluid cushion sits between the surfaces. Boosted lubrication occurs as water in the synovial fluid is forced into the cartilage, leaving behind a more concentrated fluid to lubricate the surfaces. Weeping lubrication occurs as joint loading forces synovial fluid out of the loaded cartilage and reabsorbs it in the unloaded areas.

6. C See answer to question 5.

7. C

- Fatigue wear is failure of a material after multiple cycles of load below the yield point resulting in cracking and macroscopic failure.
- Third body wear occurs when body enters between the articulating surfaces.
- Adhesive wear occurs due to hydrogen bonds, resulting in the weaker bearing surface being torn off with contact sheer forces.
- Abrasive wear is due to a harder material eroding the surface of a softer material
- Backside wear occurs when two non-articulating surfaces rub together e.g. the back surface of a polyethylene liner and its associated acetabular shell.

Although all types of wear are possible after a total hip replacement, in a well-functioning prosthesis the main type of wear is adhesive.

8. A The linear portion of the gradient of a stress strain curve is the Young's modulus.

Material	Approximate Young's modulus (GPa)
Ceramic	350
Cobalt chrome	250
Stainless steel	190
Titanium	110
Cortical bone	20
PMMA	3
Cancellous bone	1

9. E The advantages of using a ceramic in total joint arthroplasty include:

- High strength
- High Young's modulus
- Surface hardness
- Very smooth surface
- Highly wettable (hydrophilic surface)
- Low wear
- Large head sizes possible due to low adhesive wear

Disadvantages are:

- Brittle (very short plastic region on stress-strain curve)
- Non-malleable

10. A Orthopaedic implants can be susceptible to several corrosion modes.

Galvanic corrosion occurs due to the transfer of electrons down an electrochemical gradient between two metals in physical contact with one another in the same conductive solution.

Fretting corrosion occurs due to micromotion between materials in contact when under load.

Crevice corrosion is a localized form of corrosion between a material and its local fluid environment, which has limited exchange with the larger fluid environment.

Pitting corrosion is a form of localized corrosion that results in the formation of little holes or pits. Small grain defects result in galvanic corrosion and the subsequent production of the 'pit' in which a local electrochemical environment persists and continues the corrosive process.

Stress corrosion occurs secondarily to the combined processes of corrosion and applied stress.

11. A The working length of a plate is defined as the unsupported distance across a fracture site. This is often between the two screws closest to the fracture, but may be the plate itself eg in a buttress plate.

The pitch of a screw is the axial distance between two consecutive threads. The core diameter is the diameter of the shaft of the screw. The lead is the distance advanced by the screw when it is turned one complete revolution.

The area moment of inertia is a measure of the resistance of a beam to bending around an axis lying in the cross-sectional plane.

12. A Passivation occurs when a material becomes coated in a thin layer that protects it from corrosion. Titanium is always used as an example within orthopaedics as a material that can self-passify by the formation of a titanium oxide coat. Stainless steel is more resistant to corrosion than iron but it can still rust. It can be passified by a number of different chemical processes but does not self-passify.

13. B Screw pullout strength is dependent upon diameter of the thread and the diameter of the core. Screw thread pitch and depth both influence pullout strength and are interrelated by the 'thread area'. The pullout strength of a screw is determined by the total thread area.

The following will increase resistance to pullout:
- Decreasing thread pitch
- Decreasing core diameter
- Increasing thread depth (particularly in porous materials).
- Cannulation in isolation does not influence screw pull out strength, but decreases the strength of the screw and tends to increase core diameter.

14. A Fatigue failure is probably the commonest mode of failure of orthopaedic implants.

The endurance limit is the stress at which a specimen can withstand an infinite number of cyclical loads without failing. As this is difficult to measure it is arbitrarily defined as the maximum stress at which a material can withstand ten million cycles. It is plotted on a stress (S) to number of cycles (N) curve, or S-N curve. Above this value the applied stress and the number of cycles that can be withstood are inversely related.

Yield strength is the lowest stress at which permanent (plastic) deformation occurs.

The elastic limit is the maximum stress that can be applied before a material undergoes permanent deformation. Up to this value removal of the stress will allow the material to return to its original shape. This is marked by the end of the linear portion of the stress-strain curve. (A loose synonym is yield strength).

Breaking stress is the stress at which fracture of the material occurs.

The area under the stress-strain curve at any point is a measure of the total energy per unit volume that has been used to reach the point on the curve.

15. E A viscoelastic material possesses the following properties:

Creep – the continued deformation of a material over time in response to an applied stress

Hysteresis is seen as the difference in the shape of the loading and unloading curve, and often resembling a loop. The area between the loading and unloading curves is the energy 'lost' as heat by going from loading to unloading

Strain rate dependency – the Young's modulus depends upon the rate at which the stress is applied.

Stress relaxation – in response to a constantly applied strain the stress experienced by the material decreases

Wear resistance is not a property of viscoelastic materials. It is more related to surface hardness.

16. **B** Metal implants can be manufactured by casting, forging or extrusion. After the initial process their material properties can be altered by additional steps, such as cold working or annealing.

Casting involves pouring a molten metal into a mould and allowing it to cool. The rate of cooling affects the eventual grain size and therefore the material properties.

Forging involves forcing a material into a mould. This can be conducted at hot, warm or cold temperatures.

Annealing involves heating the material to just below melting point with subsequent cooling. The eventual grain size is determined by the peak temperature and rate of cooling.

Cold working (also known as strain hardening or work hardening) is the plastic deformation of a material at a temperature below its crystallisation point. It induces dislocations and decreases grain size within the material which in turn leads to improvements in strength.

17. **D** Solid PMMA is formed by mixing a powder and a liquid. The powder is polymerised PMMA and contains an initiator, dibenzoyl peroxide and a radio opacifier, either Barium sulphate ($BaSO_4$) or zirconia (ZrO_2). The liquid is mainly methylmethacrylate monomer with added hydroquinone and N,N-dimethyl-*p*-toluidine. Hydroquinone inhibits polymerization of the liquid before its addition to the powder. Polymerisation begins when the liquid contacts the dibenzoyl peroxide. The N,N-dimethyl-*p*-toluidine then accelerates polymerization once the reaction begins.

18. **C** Phase transformation has been reported to be a concern with zirconia ceramic. It does not occur with alumina. The crystal structure has been reported to be unstable at body temperature in vitro and this has been reported to lead to premature failure in the body. This has limited its use within orthopaedics.

K. Haraguchi et al. Phase transformation of a zirconia ceramic head after total hip arthroplasty. JBJS Br 2001; 83–B:996–1000

19.   A   The only material present in the list that is commonly affected by galvanic corrosion in the body is cobalt chrome. Titanium is never present in its pure form and is more usually present in oxide forms often with aluminium. Titanium alloys can undergo galvanic corrosion either when mated to stainless steel screws or when used in locking plates which disrupt the protective oxide layer (commonly called cold welding). Titanium galvanic corrosion is commonly clinically seen as the 'black' staining seen in tissues surrounding previously implanted titanium alloy implants.

20.   B   Osteolysis around total joint arthroplasty is caused by activated macrophages which have been stimulated by UHMWPE particles. Over 90% of particles produced by wear of THR are less than 10μm, with an average diameter of 0.5μm. Particles between 0.1 and 1μm are the most biologically active; those larger than 10μm are not easily ingested by macrophages.

Campbell P, et al. Isolation of predominantly submicron-sized UHMWPE wear particles from periprosthetic tissues. J Biomed Mater Res 1995, 29:127–31

21.   E   Particles within the size range 0.1–1.0μm are the most biologically active. Particles implicated in osteolysis can come from any part of the total arthroplasty system, e.g. UHMWPE, metals, ceramic, cement, if they are the correct size. Some materials are more biologically active than others. The activity of macrophages is dependent upon the dose of biologically active particles released. All of the features mentioned above are important in the generation of osteolysis.

Extending Matching Answers

1. **A** Creep is continued deformation under an applied load. It is a property of viscoelastic materials and is both temperature and time dependent.

2. **C** The resistance of a structure to deformation is called the stiffness. Stiffness is not the same as Young's modulus. The stiffness is both material and structure dependent, whereas Young's modulus is an inherent property of the material. (In orthopaedics they are often used interchangeably.)

Young's modulus is the gradient of the stress-strain curve in the elastic region.

3. **D** Strain is change in length divided by the initial length in response to an applied stress. It is dimensionless (although it is sometimes expressed as a percentage).

4. **E** Stress – a measure of force applied per unit area. Expressed is N/m^2, or Pascals.

5. **G** The strength of a material is defined as the ability of a material to withstand an applied stress without failing. There are a number of confusing terms that use terms interchangeably.

True elastic limit

The lowest stress at which irrevocable molecular movement occurs.

Offset yield point (proof stress)

As a yield point is difficult to determine, engineers frequently use an arbitrary point of 0.1 or 0.2% of the strain as the offset yield point on the stress strain curve.

Proportional limit is the stress at which the linear portion of the stress-strain curve ends.

6. **F** Stress relaxation is the decrease in stress in a body over the application of a constant strain.

7. **D** The mechanical properties of both tantalum and titanium are sensitive to surface flaws – notch sensitivity.

8. C Alumina ceramic is a monophasic polycrystalline ceramic. Alumina is has an ionic structure that creates a hydrophilic surface. This results in wettability greater than polyethylene or cobalt chrome and helps to generate fluid-film. The hardness of alumina means that the bearing surface is very smooth and has a high scratch resistance. These qualities mean that there is a reduction of abrasive wear and third body wear. The wettability allows for greater lubrication and a reduction in adhesive wear compared to metal on polyethylene bearings.

9. E The highly reactive chromium ions undergo sacrificial protection and stabilise the ferrous component of stainless steel preventing oxidisation.

10. G Stainless steels contain sufficient chromium to form a passive film of chromium oxide, which prevents further surface corrosion and blocks corrosion from spreading into the metal's internal structure.

Surgical stainless steel is a specific type of stainless steel, used in medical applications. It is composed of chromium, nickel and molybdenum. The alloy used in joint replacement is 316L. The 'L' means that the carbon content of the alloy is low, i.e. below 0.03%. The chromium gives the metal scratch and corrosion resistance. The steel exhibits great resistance to chloride pitting and crevice corrosion and increased hardness because of high molybdenum content (>6%) and the nickel content ensures better resistance to stress-corrosion.

11. F Vanadium stabilizes titanium and increases its strength and temperature stability. It is commonly used with aluminium to produce the alloy titanium 6Al-4V, which contains 6% aluminium and 4% vanadium.

12. D Tantalum, atomic number 73, has a trabecular structure which is 100 % interconnected with a porosity of 80%; this contributes to its excellent biocompatibility and potential for osteointergration. Its modulus is very similar to cancellous bone. It can be used for uncemented joint replacement reconstruction.

13. C Hot isostatic pressing (HIP) is a manufacturing process used to increase the density of the ceramic materials and improve the grain size. The HIP process subjects a component to both elevated temperature and high gas pressure in a containment vessel.

Chapter 9

Gait, Prosthetics, Foot and Ankle Biomechanics

> MCQ 20
> EMQ 15

Multiple Choice Questions

1. **Which one of the following is NOT one of the prerequisites for normal gait as described by Gage?**
    a. Adequate foot clearance during swing phase
    b. Sufficient step length
    c. Hindfoot flexibility during heel-strike
    d. Stability during stance phase
    e. Correct pre-positioning of foot immediately prior to heel-strike

2. **One step is defined as:**
    a. The distance between heel-strike with one foot and the next heel-strike on the same side
    b. The distance between heel-strike with one foot and the next heel-strike on the contralateral side
    c. The distance travelled between heel-strike with one foot and toe-off on the same side
    d. The distance travelled between heel-strike with one foot and toe-off on the contralateral side
    e. The distance between toe-off with one foot and the next heel-strike with the same foot

3. **Which of the following best describes the functional biomechanics of the ankle joint?**

    a. An *Archimedes*-type spiral screw of 12° helical orientation
    b. An *Archimedes*-type spiral screw of 15° helical orientation
    c. A hinge with axis at 7° to the horizontal, with superimposed *frustrum* resulting in broader radius of curvature laterally than medially
    d. A hinge with axis at 10° to the horizontal, with superimposed *frustrum* resulting in broader radius of curvature laterally than medially
    e. A hinge with axis at 10° to the horizontal, with superimposed *frustrum* resulting in broader radius of curvature medially than laterally

4. **Which is the correct position for fusion of the ankle joint?**

    a. Neutral rotation, neutral dorsi-/plantarflexion, neutral varus/valgus
    b. 5° external rotation, neutral dorsi-/plantarflexion, 5° valgus
    c. Neutral rotation, neutral dorsi-/plantarflexion, 5° varus
    d. 5° external rotation, 5° dorsiflexion, 5° varus
    e. 5° external rotation, 5° dorsiflexion, neutral varus/valgus

5. **What is the approximate increase in energy requirement for walking following above knee amputation?**

    a. 35%
    b. 45%
    c. 55%
    d. 65%
    e. 75%

6. **Which of the following is NOT a feature of the second 'rocker' (interval) phase of stance during the gait cycle?**

    a. Contraction of tibialis anterior
    b. Contraction of tibialis posterior
    c. Contraction of peroneus longus
    d. Contraction of peroneus brevis
    e. Contraction of gastrocsoleus complex

7. **What clinical entity is assessed by the Coleman block test?**

    a. Whether first ray flexion is fixed or flexible
    b. Whether hindfoot varus is fixed or flexible
    c. Whether forefoot adduction is fixed or flexible
    d. Whether 1st MTP joint abduction is fixed or flexible
    e. Whether midfoot equinus is fixed or flexible

8. **Which one of the following changes would be expected to be seen in the gait cycle following loss of function of the right hip abductors?**

    a. Increased circumduction of right hip during swing phase
    b. Increased upward pelvic tilt during left stance phase
    c. Increased dorsiflexion of right ankle during swing phase
    d. Increased flexion of left knee during swing phase
    e. Increased plantarflexion of right ankle during swing phase

9. **Which of the following is most likely to lead to prosthesis pistoning during the swing phase in the below-knee amputee?**

    a. Poorly functioning suspension system
    b. Poor socket fit
    c. Excessive prosthesis length
    d. Insufficient prosthesis length
    e. Plantarflexed foot

10. **The Scott-Craig orthosis is a specialised type of:**

    a. Foot-orthosis
    b. Ankle-foot orthosis
    c. Knee-ankle-foot orthosis
    d. Hip-knee-ankle-foot orthosis
    e. Trunk-hip-knee-ankle-foot orthosis

11. **Which of the following statements regarding the stance phase of gait is TRUE?**

    a. Inadequate function in the soleus muscle may manifest as prolonged knee flexion during late stance
    b. Posterior trunk lean in midstance may be a sign of fixed plantarflexion of the ankle
    c. During midstance the ground reaction force is posterior to the knee
    d. Fixed plantarflexion of the ankle characteristically results in increased knee flexion throughout stance
    e. The average flexion in the hip at the time of initial contact is 20°

12. **Which of the following is the correct definition of biological amputation level?**

    a. The most distal level at which neurological function is completely normal
    b. The most distal level at which amputation will support normal wound healing
    c. The most distal level at which any trace of either sensory or motor function is detectable
    d. The most proximal level at which a joint-sparing amputation can be undertaken
    e. The most proximal level at which amputation may be undertaken without leading to loss of independent mobilisation

13. **Which of the following statements regarding the transverse tarsal joints is FALSE?**

    a. The talonavicular and calcaneocuboid joints adopt parallel alignment when the foot is in pronation
    b. The transverse tarsal joints are best able to adapt to uneven ground when the hindfoot is in varus
    c. The transverse tarsal joints become increasingly divergent immediately prior to toe-off
    d. The superior axes of both Chopart joints pass through the neck of the talus
    e. The talonavicular joint is a ball-and-socket joint

14. **Which of the following correctly describes the University of California at Berkeley Laboratory (UCBL) insert?**

    a. A soft elastofoam insert encompassing the hind-foot used in the symptomatic treatment of plantar fasciitis
    b. A soft elastofoam insert encompassing the hind- and midfoot used in the symptomatic treatment of plantar fasciitis and pes planus
    c. A rigid plastic insert encompassing the hind-foot to control heel valgus
    d. A rigid plastic insert encompassing the mid- and fore-foot to re-disperse the forces that contribute to transfer metatarsalgia
    e. A rigid plastic insert encompassing the hind- and mid-foot to control hindfoot valgus and midfoot pronation

15. **What is the most appropriate functional application of a Ground Reaction ankle-foot orthosis?**

    a. Create a flexion moment at the knee to prevent hyperextension in patients with gastrocsoleus dysfunction
    b. Prevent foot drop during the initial loading phase in patients with weak dorsiflexors
    c. Limit flexion moment at the hip to avoid excessive pelvic tilt in patients with weak hip and knee extensors
    d. Create an extension moment at the knee to prevent excessive flexion in patients with quadriceps dysfunction
    e. Prevent plantarflexion, varus or valgus deviation whilst allowing dorsiflexion in cerebral palsy patients with low ICF scores

16. **Which of the following occurs during the initial contact phase of the gait cycle?**

    a. Forefoot supination
    b. Eccentric loading of the medial portion of the Achilles' tendon
    c. Isometric contraction of the hip flexors
    d. Eccentric contraction of the gastrocsoleus complex
    e. Concentric contraction of tibialis anterior

17. Which of the following statements regarding the metatarsal break is TRUE?

a. In the normal adult population the metatarsal break ranges from 30–50°

b. An effect of the metatarsal break is to cause pronation of the foot during terminal stance

c. The metatarsal break is also referred to in some textbooks as a 'march fracture'

d. The metatarsal break results from the fact that the first metatarsal is the longest of the five metatarsal bones

e. The metatarsal break is a contributory factor to the steady tightening in the plantar fascia during terminal stance

18. Which of the following does NOT occur when the metatarsophalangeal joints are extended?

a. Locking of the midtarsal joints

b. Locking of the transverse tarsal joint

c. Increased varus position of the os calcis

d. Increased distance between os calcis and metatarsal heads

e. Increased tension in the plantar fascia

19. Which of the following statements regarding the subtalar joint is FALSE?

a. In the normal foot the mean functional range of subtalar movement during the gait cycle is 6°

b. As the hindfoot is everted the os calcis moves anteriorly

c. The axis of subtalar rotation is 16° and 42° in the transverse and sagittal planes respectively

d. A given degree of tibial torsion has an increased rotatory effect on foot position in flatfooted individuals

e. The maximum achievable range of passive inversion in the non-diseased subtalar joint is 20°

20. **What proportion of the total gait cycle would be expected to be occupied by the double stance phase in a healthy 25-year-old male?**

    a. 10%
    b. 14%
    c. 18%
    d. 22%
    e. 26%

Extended Matching Questions

SCENARIO I OPTIONS

A Friction varies with degree of flexion

B Relatively limited stability during stance

C Weight activated braking of the hinge mechanism

D Moveable axis of flexion

E Slowing of movement during swing phase and into knee extension

F Energy is stored in spring mechanism prior to toe-off

G Complete stability during stance phase/standing

H Increase in number of steps per minute increases friction

This question concerns the different types of knee articulation mechanisms that may be employed in lower limb prostheses. For each of the following types of articulation, select the feature from the list above that most accurately describes its mode of action. Each option may be used once, more than once or not at all; however, for each question there is only one correct answer from the list.

1. Manual locking knee

2. Constant friction knee

3. Hydraulic swing phase control knee

4. Stance control knee

5. Polycentric knee

SCENARIO II OPTIONS

A Medial heel wedge
B Lateral heel wedge
C Metatarsal dome insole
D Metatarsal bar
E Box shoe with midfoot plantar recess
F Rocker bottom shoe

G Carbon-fibre ankle-foot orthosis
H Jointed ankle-foot orthosis with inferior spring
I Rigid ankle-foot orthosis
J Rigid knee-ankle-foot orthosis

Above is a list of different types of orthoses used around the lower limb. For each of the clinical presentations below, select the most appropriate orthosis. Each option may be used once, more than once or not at all.

6. A 50-year-old female presents with a painful Morton's neuroma. She does not wish to undergo surgery.

7. A 38-year-old male complains of chronic post-traumatic dysfunction of the gastrocsoleus complex. No other muscle groups are affected.

8. A 69-year-old presents with flaccid paralysis affecting all muscle groups below the knee.

9. A 72-year-old female requires symptomatic control of her tarsometatarsal osteoarthritis.

10. A 48-year-old diabetic with established Charcot's foot is starting to develop a pressure ulcer over the medial aspect of the sole of the foot.

SCENARIO III OPTIONS

A Heel too soft   **F** Knee too stiff

B Heel too hard   **G** Knee not stiff enough

C Heel too stiff   **H** Knee too anterior

D Prosthesis too long   **I** Knee too varus

E Prosthesis too short   **J** Knee too posterior

Above is a list of possible technical faults that may occur following prosthesis fitting for above knee amputation. For each of the gait abnormalities listed below, select the most likely cause from the list. Each option may be used once, more than once or not at all.

11. Foot slapdown

12. Medial 'whip'

13. Foot rotates during initial contact phase

14. Shortened duration of stance phase

15. Vaulted gait

Answers: Chapter 9

MCQ 20
EMQ 15

Multiple Choice Answers

1. C Gage has identified five prerequisites which must be met in order for normal gait to exist. (*Gage. Clin Dev Med* 1991). They are:
- Stability during stance phase
- Sufficient step length
- Adequate foot clearance during swing phase
- Correct foot pre-positioning immediately prior to heel-strike
- Conservation of energy throughout gait cycle

2. B *Step length* is the horizontal distance covered between heel-strike with one foot and the next heel-strike with the contralateral foot.

Stride length is the horizontal distance covered between heel-strike with one foot and the next heel-strike with the same foot.

Cadence is the number of steps taken per minute.

3. D The ankle joint is effectively a hinge joint with its line of axis running between the tips of the medial and lateral malleoli, such that its angle is oblique by 10°. However, the dome of the talus is wider anteriorly than posteriorly. The articular surfaces on both tibial and talar sides are such that a shape formed said to be part of the *frustrum* of a cone whose apex is located to the medial side of the ankle joint. The net result of these structural features causes the forefoot to move from a relatively abducted position to an adducted one as the ankle moves from dorsiflexion to plantarflexion. The fibula externally rotates as the ankle dorsiflexes to accommodate the wider anterior portion of the talus.

The Archimedes screw analogy is one applied to the subtalar, not ankle joint.

4. B   It is impossible to fuse the ankle in such a way that the gait cycle is not in any way affected; the best compromise is 5°–10° external rotation, neutral dorsi-/plantarflexion and 5° valgus. This still tends to result in a reduced duration of the first and second rockers, with the third being less affected. The position allows for the most normal foot progression angle, subtalar loading and foot pre-positioning. There is inevitably a compensatory increase in movement at other joints in the hindfoot, although in time this may result in arthritic changes in these joints.

5. D   The increase in energy requirements for walking is often a key determinant of long-term functional outcome following amputation, and if at all possible should be borne in mind when planning the level of transection. A number of authors have attempted to quantify the increase in requirement following transection at different levels:

Transection level	% increase in energy for walking
Low below-knee	10
Average below-knee	25
High below-knee	40
Above knee	60–70
Hip disarticulation	100–150
Hindquarter	150–200

Bilateral amputation results in increased energy requirements that are significantly more than twice that of unilateral surgery.

6. A   The stance phase of the gait cycle may be subdivided into three intervals or 'rockers'; the first describes the segment between heel-strike and the foot coming fully into contact with the ground (foot flat); the second is the period during which the entire plantar aspect of the foot is full contact; the third refers to the pre-swing period during which the toes and metatarsal heads remain in contact, but the hindfoot is lifting up.

During the second rocker, the centre of gravity moves forward from a position behind the ankle to one in front, with a resultant passive dorsiflexion of the ankle – eccentric contraction in the gastrocsoleus complex controls this process. The subtalar joint is then inverted by contraction of tibialis posterior, creating a rigid hindfoot in the lead up to toe-off. This process is limited by simultaneous eccentric contraction of both peroneus longus and brevis; this ensures that the tibialis posterior contraction described does not occur unopposed.

7. B The Coleman block test is used in the assessment of the cavovarus foot, to demonstrate whether or not the subtalar complex is mobile and whether the deformity is being driven by the hindfoot or the first ray. The test involves placing a wooden block under the foot, but with the first toe and metatarsal head in contact with the floor – this effectively eliminates the first ray flexion. The hindfoot can then be observed to see whether the varus deformity corrects; if it does correct then the deformity is being driven by the first ray (stiff plantarflexed first ray and the hind foot is compensating); if it does not correct then the deformity is being driven by the hindfoot (stiff hindfoot and the first ray is plantarflexing to compensate).

8. D The loss of right hip abductor function will cause a Trendelenburg gait, such that the pelvis tilts to the floor during the right-sided stance phase. This creates a functional leg-length discrepancy such that the right is effectively shorter than the left. Several strategies are available during left-sided swing phase to overcome this problem – often more than one will be used in conjunction:

- Increased left-sided ankle dorsiflexion
- Increased left-sided knee flexion
- Increased left-sided hip circumduction

The fourth strategy for overcoming a leg-length discrepancy is to increase upward pelvic tilt when the shorter side is in stance phase; but in the case described here this clearly not possible due to the loss of abductor function.

9. A Inadequate functioning in the suspension mechanism can characteristically cause a below knee prosthesis to piston during the swing phase of gait. Conversely, pistoning during stance is more likely to result from poor fit of the prosthesis onto the stump. Incorrect length will lead to the usual gait features seen in any patient with a leg length discrepancy (see question 8). Plantarflexion of the prosthetic foot can cause an increase in patellar pressure.

10. C The Scott-Craig knee-ankle-foot orthosis is most commonly used in paraplegic patients following injury to the spinal cord. A solid base of support is provided by the combination of a reinforced shoe and a fixed ankle, with adjustable supports such that the ankle position can be altered. The aim is to lock the ankle in slight dorsiflexion; the knee is also fixed and the patient can then be taught to mobilise independently by leaning back with the hips in a mild degree of extension, relying on the iliofemoral ligaments to prevent hyperextension. This technique is not suitable for use in paediatric patients as the iliofemoral ligaments are not fully developed until adolescence.

11 A Soleal weakness characteristically leads to both delayed heel-rise in terminal stance and to prolonged flexion of the knee at the same time, as the extensor mechanism does not have a stable construct against which to work. At the time of initial contact, average flexion in the hip is 35°. At heel-strike the ground reaction force (GRF) is posterior to the knee; however, as the knee extends during midstance the GRF passes anteriorly, before moving back posteriorly again as the knee flexes during terminal stance. Fixed ankle plantarflexion results in early heelrise during midstance, as well as anterior trunk lean and hyperextension of the knee. Both of these mechanisms form part of an attempt to maintain forward progression of the GRF over the ankle during mid- and terminal stance.

12. B This terminology is used particularly in reference to amputation for peripheral vascular disease (PVD). Selection of amputation level in PVD can be challenging; a balance must be reached that allows maximum preservation of function whilst affording a realistic likelihood of wound healing, without which application of a prosthesis is not possible. The level that allows this compromise to be reached is termed the biological amputation level.

13. B   The transverse tarsal joints are central to the dual functions of the foot as flexible during the early and midstance phases of gait, whilst forming a solid construct during terminal stance. The calcaneocuboid joint (CCJ) is a saddle joint whilst the talonavicular (TNJ) is a ball-and-socket joint; both have superior axes passing through the talar neck and inferior axes that traverse the body of the os calcis. When the foot is everted and pronated in the earlier phases of stance, with the heel in varus, the alignment of the TNJ and CCJ is effectively parallel, affording the hind- and mid-foot significant flexibility and allowing adaptation to uneven ground. However, during heelrise, the os calcis swings into varus, the foot supinates and the axes of the two Chopart joints diverge, stiffening the foot as a whole; and providing the stable platform needed during preswing.

14. E   The UCBL insert is a rigid plastic shoe insert which encompasses the hind- and mid-foot to control hindfoot valgus and pronation of the midfoot.

15. D   The GRAFO has a rigid toe plate, ankle and lower calf and an anterior proximal portion that wraps firmly around the anterior tibia. It is used to transfer the ground reaction force to provide knee support for patients with weak quadriceps and gastrocsoleus function. The combination of the components of the shell means that plantarflexion is coupled with knee extension (a plantarflexion-knee extension couple (PF/KE)) causing a knee extension moment. It accentuates knee extension in midstance and places the extension moment closer to the knee. The GRAFO is rigid and therefore allows no ankle motion in any direction. (The ICF refers to the International Classification of Functioning, Disability and Health).

16. B   The Achilles' tendon undergoes eccentric loading medially during the initial contact and loading response phases of the gait cycle (first rocker), due to the pronation of the foot that occurs immediately following heelstrike. At the same time there is eccentric contraction of all muscles in the anterior compartment – this controls the passive plantarflexion occurring until midstance, and prevents 'slapdown' of the foot. The gastrocsoleus does not commence its eccentric contraction until midstance, when it has a role in controlling the transference of the ground reaction force from behind to in front of the ankle; it then moves into powerful concentric contraction during terminal stance and toe-off. The hip flexors are not active until the very end of stance as they prepare for the swing phase.

17. E The metatarsal break refers to a line drawn through the five MTP joints, the second metatarsal being the longest and the fifth being the shortest. There is considerable variation in the adult population, with the angulation of the break ranging from 50–70°. The break causes the foot to undergo a degree of supination during the terminal stance phase; the first and second MTP joints therefore extend earlier than the fourth and fifth, causing a steady tightening in the plantar fascia, and a resultant locking of the hind- and mid-foot joint via the *Spanish windlass* mechanism.

A march fracture is a distal stress fracture of one of the metatarsal shafts, and has no relation to the metatarsal break.

18. D The so-called *Spanish windlass* mechanism is one of the keys to understanding how the foot can switch between being flexible and completely rigid at different stages in the gait cycle; the mechanism stems from the attachments of the plantar fascia to the os calcis at one end and the bases of the proximal phalanges at the other. During the heel-rise portion of the stance phase, extension of the MTP joints increases the tension in the fascia, which in turn reduces the distance between the os calcis and the metatarsal heads. This simultaneously brings the os calcis into varus, locks the midtarsal joints and also, via the subtalar joint, locks the transverse tarsal joint. After toe-off the process is reversed allowing the foot to become flexible during the swing phase.

19. B Subtalar motion is somewhat complex, and is best understood by two models superimposed. The first is that of a simple *mitred hinge*; this transforms tibial rotation into pronation and supination of the foot, and would do so at a ratio of 1:1 were the hinge at 45°. In reality the axis in healthy individuals is 16° and 42° in the transverse and sagittal planes respectively, although this is altered in those with flat feet such that there is an increase in the amount of pronation/supination per degree of tibial rotation. The second model is that of an *Archimedes' screw*, which causes the os calcis to move anteriorly or posteriorly as the hindfoot is respectively either inverted or everted. The maximum range of motion in the normal subtalar joint is 5° of eversion and 20° of inversion; however, the functional range in normal walking is only 6°.

20. C Normal 'adult' gait is established by the age of 7. During each stride, the double stance phase occupies approximately 18% of the full gait cycle. In later life this steadily increases even in healthy individuals, whilst both self-selected and maximum possible walking speeds reduce from the eighth decade onwards.

Extending Matching Answers

1. G

2. B

3. E

4. C

5. D

The manual locking knee provides absolute stability but at the expense of a grossly abnormal gait, in addition to which it requires manual unlocking to allow sitting down. A constant friction joint is relatively unstable but has the advantage of allowing a fairly large range of motion. In a hydraulic swing phase control knee, deceleration during swing phase and into knee extension allows good variation in number of steps per minute, but at the expense of cost. Stance control knees effectively 'lock' when weight is transmitted across them, allowing flexibility during swing but not at the expense of stability during stance. Polycentric knees provided excellent stability in stance, whilst allowing considerable flexion when needed; however, they are costly. There is no prosthetic knee which stores energy in a spring mechanism prior to toe-off.

6. C

7. H

8. G

9. F

10. E

Foot orthoses may be provided in the form of insoles or shoes, and may be either custom made or 'off the shelf'. Ankle-foot orthoses may be rigid, semi-rigid or spring-assisted.

A metatarsal dome is similar in function to a metatarsal (MT) bar in that it supports the distal metatarsal heads immediately proximal to the MT heads. However, whereas a bar supports all five MTs, a dome usually supports only the second, third and fourth. It therefore relieves pressure between the MT heads and is thus often beneficial in relieving the pain of a Morton's neuroma.

A jointed ankle-foot orthosis with inferior spring allows a full range of movement whilst providing assistance with plantarflexion via the return of conserved energy; it is therefore ideal in assisting terminal stance and toe-off in patients in whom active plantarflexion is impaired.

A carbon fibre AFO allows movement whilst providing support, and is therefore often used in patients with flaccid paralysis in whom passive range of motion is well preserved.

A rocker bottom sole reduces flexion and extension forces in the arthritic midfoot, especially in late stance.

In Charcot's foot a custom made shoe with plantar recess under the midfoot will offload the pressure area and potentially reduce ulceration without recourse to a total contact cast. During the inflammatory phase a total contact cast is normally required but in established Charcot foot a custom shoe will often control the ulceration.

11. A

12. I

13. C

14. G

15. D

The commonest abnormalities that may occur with above knee prostheses are tabulated below, along with their likely effects on the gait cycle:

Technical fault	Gait abnormality
Heel too soft	'Slapdown' of foot
Heel too hard	Excessive flexion of knee
Heel too stiff	Foot rotates during initial contact phase
Prosthesis too long	Vaulted gait
Prosthesis too short	Lateral trunk bending
Poor socket fit	Lateral trunk bend, foot rotation during initial contact phase
Poor suspension	Vaulted gait, foot rotation during initial contact phase
Knee too stiff	Circumduction during swing phase
Knee not stiff enough	Shortened duration of stance phase
Knee too anterior	Instability of knee, excessive knee flexion during stance phase
Knee too varus	'Medial whip' (i.e. heel displaces outwards then inwards during stance)
Knee too valgus	'Lateral whip'

Chapter 10
Orthopaedic Pathology

MCQ 31
EMQ 15

Multiple Choice Questions

1. Which of the following statements concerning hypophos-phataemic rickets is FALSE?
   a. It is a rare X-linked dominant form of rickets
   b. Serum phosphate levels are decreased
   c. Calcium and PTH levels are normal
   d. Physiological 25- and 1,25-vitamin D levels are seen
   e. Treatment is with phosphate and vitamin D_3

2. With regards to gout, which of the following best describes the classical radiological and microscopic findings?
   a. Chondral calcification and negatively birefringent needle yellow crystals
   b. Perichondral 'rat's bite' cysts and negatively birefringent needle yellow crystals
   c. Chondral calcification and negatively birefringent pink crystals
   d. Perichondral 'rat's bite' cysts and positively birefringent needle yellow crystals
   e. Perichondral 'rat's bite' cysts and positively birefringent pink crystals

3. A patient presents with bowed tibia and the following biochemical picture. What is the diagnosis?

Increased: *PTH & Alk Phos*
Decreased: *Calcium, Phosphate, 25 Vit D, Urine Ca*

a. Primary hyperparathyroidism
b. Hypoparathyroidism
c. Pseudohyperparathroidism
d. Hypophosphataemic rickets
e. Vitamin D deficient rickets

4. All types of rickets have a failure at which of the following physeal zones?

a. Reserve zone
b. Proliferative zone
c. Zone of provisional calcification
d. Groove of Ranvier
E. Hypertrophic zone

5. All of the following are differences between pseudohypoparathyroidism and hypoparathyroidism EXCEPT:

a. Pseudohypoparathyroidism has a normal alkaline phosphatase, whilst hypoparathroidism does not due to parathyroid failure.
b. In pseudohypoparathyroidism PTH may be normal, whereas in hypoparathyroidism, by definition, it may not be.
c. Pseudohypoparathyroidism may be due to PTH resistance whilst primary hypoparathyroidism may not.
d. Primary hypoparathyroidism is often caused by a parathyroid adenoma; pseudohypoparathyroidism cannot be.
e. Pseudohypoparathyroidism may present with a raised PTH.

6. **With regards to osteomalacia which of the following statements is TRUE?**
    a. Osteomalacia is a quantitative disorder of bone
    b. It is often seen in association with hypercalcaemia and hyper-phosphataemia
    c. It results from mineralisation of defective matrix
    d. Osteomalacia is most commonly caused by renal osteodystrophy resulting from indigestion agents or antacids.
    e. Idiopathic transient osteoporosis may be associated with osteomalacia

7. **Osteogenesis imperfecta is always associated with all of the following EXCEPT:**
    a. A defect in collagen synthesis
    b. Blue sclerae
    c. A genetic defect which may be either heritable or a new defect
    d. A failure in the production of normal bone associated with pathological fractures
    e. Progressive tibial bowing and kyphosis

8. **Which one of the following statements regarding malignant hyperpyrexia is FALSE?**
    a. An autosomal dominant inheritance pattern is seen
    b. There are associations with Duchenne muscular dystrophy and osteogenesis imperfecta
    c. Malignant hyperpyrexia may be triggered by a range of anaesthetic agents including succinylcholine and dantrolene
    d. The net result is impaired mitochondrial function and loss of calcium homeostasis
    e. Malignant hyperpyrexia is often unrecognised and may be rapidly fatal

9. **Which of the following conditions does NOT affect the function of the reserve zone of the physis?**
   a. Achondroplasia
   b. Pseudoachondroplasia
   c. Kniest syndrome
   d. Gaucher disease
   e. Diastrophic dysplasia

10. **Which of the following conditions is NOT associated with a defect in type II collagen?**
    a. Spondyloepiphyseal dysplasia (SED)
    b. Kniest syndrome
    c. Stickler syndrome
    d. Achondroplasia
    e. Diastrophic dysplasia

11. **With regards to the proteins involved in bone and matrix regulation, which one of the following statements is INCORRECT?**
    a. Osteocalcin is manufactured by osteoblasts and production is stimulated by 1,25 vitamin D
    b. TGF-β stimulates mesenchymal stem cell differentiation into osteoblasts and has been implicated in callus formation
    c. Insulin like growth factor (IGF-1) stimulates osteocyte function
    d. Activation of the RANK receptor initiates the final common pathway in osteoclast mediated bone resorption
    e. Osteopontin functions as a cell binding protein

12. **Which one of the following statements concerning hand tumours is FALSE?**
    a. Giant cell tumours of the soft tissue and bone in the hand have similar histological appearance and can be thought of as the same entity
    b. Glomus tumours are commonly found under the nail bed and demonstrate cold intolerance
    c. Volar ganglions most commonly arise from the STT ligament
    d. Enchondromas are commonly seen at the middle phalanx
    e. Primary bone tumours are more common than metastases in the hand and wrist

13. **Which one of the following statements regarding paediatric orthopaedic oncology is TRUE?**

    a. Multiple hereditary exostoses have a small malignant potential and may transform into chondromyxoid fibroma
    b. Chondroblastoma is a painful epiphyseal lesion that abuts but rarely crosses the physis
    c. Non-ossifying fibroma (NOF) occurs normally in approximately 30% of immature skeletons
    d. The falling leaf sign is pathognomonic of a simple bone cyst
    e. Jaffe-Campanacci syndrome is characterised by large NOFs associated with mental retardation, visual problems and hirsuitism

14. **Which of the following statements concerning Ewing's Sarcoma is FALSE?**

    a. It is a malignant diaphyseal cell sarcoma affecting young patients
    b. It is associated with a chromosomal translocation 11:22 in 90% of patients
    c. It is more common than neuroblastoma in patients under the age of 5
    d. It is associated with pseudorosettes and sheets of small smudgy cells
    e. It is a primary sarcoma of bone

15. **Which of the following best describes clinical features of Hand-Schuller-Christian disease?**

    a. Affects vertebrae and long bones with typical expansile lytic lesions
    b. Punched out lesions are seen on x-ray
    c. Diffuse Langerhans cell histocytosis often fatal in the young
    d. Fluid filled lines are seen on radiographs and a bone scan shows a 'doughnut sign'
    e. Langerhans cell histocytosis affecting bone and viscera

16. **Which of the following diagnoses is NOT associated with a visible fluid level on plain radiographs?**

   a. Giant cell tumour
   b. Chondroblastoma
   c. Fibrous dysplasia
   d. Eosinophilic granuloma
   e. Simple bone cyst

17. **Which of the following statements concerning metastatic lesions of bone is FALSE?**

   a. Breast cancer frequently presents initially with metastasis to bone with no identifiable primary
   b. The valveless venous plexus of Batson accounts for the majority of metastatic tumour spread to the spine
   c. Synovial sarcoma commonly metastasises to lung
   d. Thyroid metastasis may be invisible on bone scan
   e. Benign lesions of bone cannot metastasise

18. **With reference to tumours of neural origin, which one of the following statements is FALSE?**

   a. Neurilemmoma is a benign lesion of nerve sheath and may cause symptoms by local compression; marginal excision is sufficient
   b. Neurofibromatosis may present with Lisch nodules and 'coast of California' café au lait spots
   c. Von Recklinghausen's disease is X-Linked dominant and affects 1:3000 live births
   d. Neurofibromatosis type 1 presents with bony lesions, where type 2 does not
   e. Neurofibrosarcoma may spread along the involved nerve with prolific local invasion

19. **This question concerns synovial lesions; in which of the following scenarios is the patient most likely to have a borderline malignant lesion?**

    a. A small round lesion is found near the lateral aspect of the knee which transilluminates. MRI shows a fluid filled lesion communicating with the proximal tibio-fibular joint

    b. MRI scan demonstrates diffuse nodules within the joint. Following synovectomy the histopathologist reports 'benign metaplasia' of synovial tissue

    c. Erosive changes are seen on plain radiographs both sides of the joint. MRI demonstrates high signal on T1 imaging

    d. A mass is found to arise just distal to the knee, with palpable groin lesions. X-ray demonstrates a poorly demarcated chondroid lesion

    e. Acute pain and increasing swelling are seen in the knee, which is hot red and swollen. Radiographs demonstrate calcification of both menisci and subchondral peri-articular bony erosions

20. **Which of the following is NOT a classical feature of glomus tumours?**

    a. Tumours commonly found under the nail bed

    b. Lesions represent a form of capilliary haemangioma

    c. Tumour characteristically presents as a blueish colour lesion

    d. Symptoms respond well to paracetamol

    e. Patients report cold intolerance

21. **A common finding of malignant bone and soft tissue lesions is mineralisation; in which of the following conditions is calcification NOT characteristically seen?**

    a. Synovial cell sarcoma

    b. Myeloma

    c. Liposarcoma

    d. Schwannoma

    e. Neurofibrosarcoma

22. **Which of the following lesions of bone has the lowest malignant potential?**
    a. Ollier's disease
    b. Osteochondroma
    c. Enchondroma
    d. Paget's disease
    e. Maffucci's syndrome

23. **Which of the following lesions may result following malignant pagetoid transformation?**
    a. Chondrosarcoma
    b. 'Classic' osteosarcoma
    c. Parosteal osteosarcoma
    d. Adamantinoma
    e. McCune-Albright disease

24. **Which one of the following best describes the presenting features of Hunter syndrome?**
    a. Delayed development with dermatan sulphate in urine; seen more frequently in males
    b. Delayed development with dermatan sulphate in urine; seen more frequently in females
    c. Normal development with dermatan sulphate in urine; seen more frequently in males
    d. Normal development with dermatan sulphate in urine; seen more frequently in females
    e. Normal development with keratan sulphate in urine

25. **Which of the following statements concerning dwarfism is TRUE?**
    a. Achondroplasia is a rhizomelic form of dwarfism
    b. Pseudoachondroplasia is a mesomelic form of dwarfism
    c. Achondroplastics are prone to degenerative joint disease
    d. Spondyloepiphyseal dysplasia is a form of achondroplasia
    e. Pseudoachondroplastics are prone to frontal bossing

26. **Which of the following is the most accurate description of Trevor's disease?**
    a. Single or multiple epiphyseal osteochondromata
    b. Multiple epiphyseal dysplasia
    c. Multiple epiphyseal enchondromata
    d. Autosomal dominant paediatric mucopolysaccharidosis
    e. Spondylometaphyseal dysplasia

27. **Which of the following statements concerning multiple epiphyseal dysplasia (MED) is FALSE?**
    a. MED presents as a short-limbed disproportionate dwarfism
    b. Irregular epiphyseal ossification is characteristic
    c. The severe form is known as Fairbank's disease
    d. MED has normal expression of COL IX and COMP
    e. Patients may present late with a waddling gait

28. **Which of the following statements regarding Blount's disease is TRUE?**
    a. The adolescent form is commoner than the infantile
    b. Unilateral presentation is more likely in infantile than adolescent Blount's
    c. Surgical intervention is almost always required in Langinskiold stage III and IV cases
    d. A Drennan angle of over 12° is considered abnormal
    e. Metaphyseal beaking is characteristically seen on x-ray

29. **Talipes equinovarus is associated with all of the following EXCEPT:**
    a. Larsen's disease
    b. Arthrogryposis
    c. Myelodysplasia
    d. DDH
    e. Female sex

30. **Slipped upper capital femoral epiphysis is associated with all of the following EXCEPT:**
    a. A break in Klein's line
    b. Trethowan's sign
    c. Obesity
    d. Fracture through the proliferative zone of the physis
    e. Thyroid disorders

31. **A patient presents with radial club hand. Which of the following is NOT a common association?**
    a. TAR syndrome
    b. VACTERL
    c. Fanconi's anaemia
    d. Transverse failure of formation
    e. Holt-Oram syndrome

Extended Matching Questions

SCENARIO I OPTIONS

A Undertake FRAX scoring
B Begin first-line bisphosphonate therapy
C Begin calcium therapy,
weight gain and dietary
advice

D Begin strontium therapy
E Discontinue bisphosphonate
therapy
F Undertake a DEXA scan
G Undertake a CT scan

Above is a list of possible strategies in the prevention of osteo-porosis. For each of the following clinical scenarios select the most appropriate intervention from the list. Each option may be used once, more than once or not at all.

1. A 79-year-old single lady who after a mechanical fall sustained a fractured neck of femur.

2. A 52-year-old taking HRT who trips onto an outstretched hand. Although she has no fracture the radiologist comments 'cortical osteopaenia'.

3. A 49-year-old with known osteoporosis secondary to bilateral salpingo-oopherectomy. She developed jaw pain following commencement of bisphosphonate therapy, so subsequently discontinued it herself. Her T score is -3.4 and her Z score -4.3.

SCENARIO II OPTIONS

A X linked recessive
B X linked dominant
C Autosomal recessive
D Autosomal dominant

E Mitochondrial inheritance
F Co-dominant inheritance
G Non genetic in nature

The list above describes various possible genetic inheritance patterns. Based on the clinical information given in the following cases, select the most likely pattern from the list in each case. Each option may be used once, more than once or not at all.

4. A patient has a short disproportionate stature with normal facies. He tells you he has painful knees which appear to be in a windswept posture.

5. The patient is a proportionate dwarf. He has previously had cleft palate surgery and also has a degree of kyphoscoliosis.

6. The patient describes having had bilateral Perthes' disease as a child. He is currently under investigation for a mass in his abdomen.

SCENARIO III OPTIONS

A Osteoid osteoma   **E** Enchondroma
B Osteoblastoma   **F** Osteochondroma
C Enostosis   **G** Chondromyxoid fibroma
D Myositis ossificans

This question concerns benign lesions of bone. For each of the following clinical vignettes, select the most likely diagnosis from the list above. Each option may be used once, more than once or not at all.

7. A patient complains of pain in the midfoot which responds well to NSAIDs. Plain films show a small lesion comprising ring-like sclerosis with a darker nidus in the centre.

8. A patient presents with a painful palpable lump in her buttock, deep to the subcutaneous tissue. She denies any systemic symptoms, but does recall falling from a horse 9 months previously. Radiographs demonstrate a well demarcated lesion in the gluteal area with rim calcification.

9. A 20-year-old male twists his ankle playing football and attends his general practitioner. An x-ray is obtained, which is reported as 'No fracture seen, well demarcated calcific lesion with no cortical reaction is seen in the tibial metaphysis'. Concerned, the GP arranges a bone scan which shows a 'cold' lesion.

SCENARIO IV OPTIONS

A Chondroblastoma
B Clear cell chondrosarcoma
C Intramedullary chondrosar-
coma

D Intramedullary osteosarcoma
E Telangiectatic osteosarcoma
F Parosteal osteosarcoma
G Periosteal osteosarcoma

This question concerns malignant lesions of bone. For each of the following clinical vignettes, select the most likely diagnosis from the list above. Each option may be used once, more than once or not at all.

10. A patient presents to the GP with an ulnar sided aneurysmal bone cyst of the distal radius, and is referred from their GP with radiographs showing a spreading lytic lesion with minimal mineralisation of the lesion. Bone scanning demonstrates a 'doughnut sign'.

11. A 67-year-old patient presents with hip pain and a well demarcated epiphyseal lesion of the proximal femur. MRI scanning suggests a chondroid lesion.

12. A 12-year-old girl presents with a painful knee. Radiographs demonstrate a lesion of the epiphysis crossing the physis.

SCENARIO V OPTIONS

A Groove of Ranvier
B Resting/reserve zone
C Proliferative zone
D Hypertrophic (maturation) zone

E Zone of provisional calcification
F Metaphysis
G Perichondral ring of Lacroix

Above is a list of anatomical locations within the long bones. For each of the following clinical vignettes, select the site most likely to be affected from the list. Each option may be used once, more than once or not at all.

13. During haematogenous bacterial spread and establishment of osteomyelitis or septic arthritis, which is the first region to become infected?

14. When Salter-Harris type I fracture occurs, the fracture line cleaves though this zone.

15. This is the site at which new chondrocytes are 'fed' into the growth plate from mesenchymal stem cells; it can be damaged during fractures.

Answers: Chapter 10

MCQ 31
EMQ 15

Multiple Choice Answers

1. A Hypophosphataemic vitamin D resistant rickets (or 'phosphate diabetes') is X-linked dominant; however, it is the most common form of rickets, not a rare form. The other statements are all correct.

2. B Gout is characterised by perichondral 'rat's bite' bone loss and advanced articular destruction. Needle yellow monosodium urate crystals are found within the joint; these show strong negative birefringence on microscopy with polarised light. By contrast, pseudogout classically presents with short blue weakly positively birefringent rhomboid crystals of calcium pyrophosphate, with associated chondral calcinosis.

3. E The biochemical picture is one of vitamin D deficiency rickets with secondary increase in PTH. Alkaline phosphatase levels are secondarily low due to low calcium.

4. C Rickets of all types is associated with a failure of mineralisation of normal matrix; hence it is a defect specific to the zone of provisional calcification. Hypertrophic zone would be the correct answer if there were not a more specific answer.

5. A Hypoparathyroidism and pseudohyperparathyroidism both exhibit normal alkaline phosphatase levels. PTH is raised or normal in pseudohypoparathyroidism but not in hypoparathyroidism.

6. D Renal osteodystrophy is the most common cause of osteomalacia, through the use of aluminium-containing antacids, which bind phosphate and prevent its resorption in the nephron. Osteomalacia is a qualitative disorder of bone; the matrix itself is normal.

7. B All of the other criteria are pathognomonic of osteogenesis imperfecta. The Sillence classification has been extended to include many subtypes, but postgraduate orthopaedic examination candidates are expected to know the initial four subtypes:

Type	Inheritance	Clinical features
I	Autosomal dominant	Mild with blue sclerae
II	Autosomal recessive	Extreme fragility of connective tissue, multiple *in utero* fractures, fatal. Blue sclerae
III	Autosomal recessive	Normal sclerae Extreme short stature, early onset scoliosis and in utero fracture
IV	Autosomal dominant	Normal sclerae. Later onset progressive fragility fractures. More severe than type 1.

8. C Malignant hyperpyrexia is thought to be caused by mitochondrial dysfunction, which results in a failure of calcium homeostasis. It may be triggered by a range of anaesthetic agents including halothane, and is particularly associated with osteogenesis imperfecta and the muscular dystrophies. Treatment is with intravenous dantrolene.

9. A Achondroplasia affects the proliferative zone of the physis. All the other diseases listed affect the reserve zone.

10. D Achondroplasia is associated with a defect in the receptor for FGF-3 (FGFR-3). Pseudoachondroplasia is associated with a defect in COMP. SED, diastrophic dysplasia, Kniest and Stickler syndromes are associated with defects in the COL II genes.

11. C All the statements are true excepting the function of IGF-1, which has a range of functions, but specifically stimulates matrix formation and the deposition of type I (bone) collagen.

12. A Giant cell tumours of the tendon sheath and bone share common histological features, but are completely different entities. The remaining statements are all correct.

13. C Chondroblastoma is one of the only paediatric oncology lesions that will cross an unfused physis; this is thought to be due to its origin as a chondral lesion. (The others are reported to be giant cell tumour and clear cell chondrosarcoma). Jaffe-Campanacci syndrome comprises multiple NOFs associated with café-au-lait spots, visual problems and mental retardation. NOFs are seen in 30% of normal skeletons. Although the falling leaf sign may be seen with a simple bone cyst it is not pathognomonic.

14. C Ewing's sarcoma is rare under five years of age, with neuroblastoma being considerably more common. This is an important differential diagnosis, as histologically both tumours look very similar. The other statements are all correct.

15. E Hand-Schuller-Christian disease comprises eosinophilic granulomata affecting bone and viscera. Answers A and D are both typical of aneurysmal bone cysts. An eosinophilic granuloma often appears as a punched out lesion on x-ray (answer B), whilst the diffuse Langerhans cell histocytosis described in C is the hallmark of Letterer-Siwe disease.

16. D Eosinophilic granuloma is chacracteristically associated with 'punched out' lesions on plain radiographs; the other four lesions may present with 'fluid-fluid' levels visible on plain radiographs.

17. E Giant cell tumours and chondroblastomas are both classified as benign, yet may undergo metastatic spread, with a predilection for the lung.

18. C Von Recklinghausen's disease (neurofibromatosis) is autosomal dominant; the remaining statements are all true. Lisch nodules of the iris affect the vast majority of patients over the age of 6 who present with von Recklinghausen's disease. The characteristic bone lesions are pseudoarthrosis, hypoplasia of the sphenoid wing and kyphoscoliosis. The 'smooth coast of California' café-au-lait spots help to discern the condition from McCune-Albright syndrome, in which less smooth 'coast of Maine' spots are seen. NF-2 does not have any classical bony manifestations.

19. C The scenario in C describes PVNS which may occasionally undergo malignant change; the signal change is due to haemosiderin deposition. The other scenarios described are:

A – ganglion cyst; B – synovial chondromatosis; D – chondrosarcoma; E – pseudogout

20. D Patients with glomus tumours characteristically report pinpoint tenderness that is often not relieved by simple analgesia; the other features described are all classical presenting features.

21. B The lesions described are all malignant; however, myeloma classically presents with diffuse well circumscribed lytic, rather than sclerotic lesions ('pepper-pot skull').

22. C An isolated enchondroma is not recognised as a premalignant lesion and can be managed non-operatively without long-term follow-up unless symptomatic. However, multiple enchondromas (Ollier's) lead to the development of chondrosarcoma in 20–30% of patients; this figure rises to over 90% in the presence of concurrent multiple haemangiomas (Maffucci's). Solitary osteochondromas have a less than 1% chance of progression to malignancy, as does Paget's disease (this figure is higher in patients with polyostotic Paget's).

23. B Pagetoid osteosarcoma is signalled by pain, occurs in up to 15% of patients with polyostotic Paget's and has a dismal prognosis due to its high grade (5 year survival <5%). McCune-Albright disease comprises the trio of precocious puberty (and other endocrine abnormalities), polyostotic fibrous dysplasia and café-au-lait spots.

24. A Morquio's syndrome is the only mucopolysaccharidosis with normal intelligence levels. A summary of the mucopolysaccharidoses is given below.

Type	Name	Inheritance	Development	Urinary Excretion
1	Hurler's syndrome	Autosomal recessive	Delayed	Dermatan/heparan
2	Hunter's syndrome	X-linked recessive	Delayed	Dermatan/heparan
3	Sanfilippo's syndrome	Autosomal recessive	Delayed	Heparan
4	Morquio's syndrome	Autosomal recessive	Normal	Keratan sulphate

25. **A**   Achondroplasia is a short limbed (rhizomelic) dwarfism. The following summarises some of the features of these three dwarfisms:

Characteristic	Achondroplasia	Pseudoachondroplasia	Spondyloepiphyseal Dysplasia
Appearance	Rhizomelic (short limbed)	Rhizomelic (short limbed)	Proportionate
Gene affected	FGFR-3	COMP	Congenita COL-II Tarda SEDL
Heritance	AD	AD	Congenita AD Tarda X-linked
Facies	Abnormal (frontal bossing)	Normal	Abnormal (cleft palate etc.)
Predisposition to degenerative joint disease	None	Prone	Prone

26. **A**   Trevor's disease, also known as dysplasia epiphysealis hemimelica, presents with single or multiple epiphyseal osteochondromata. Joints that may be affected include the knee, ankle or interphalangeal joints of the hands and feet.

27. **D**   The genetic basis for MED is a mutation to either COL IX (COL 9) or COMP; this results in abnormal tissue expression of the genes. All the other statements are true – the milder form is known Ribbing's disease. Radiologically MED has a similar appearance to Perthes' disease, but is bilateral.

28. **E**   Blount's disease exists in two forms – infantile and adolescent – the former being more common. The infantile is more likely to be bilateral, and is characterised by varus angulation of the proximal tibia, usually with concurrent internal tibial torsion. A Drennan angle of over 16° is considered abnormal (this is the angle between the longitudinal axis of the tibia and a line drawn through the metaphyseal beaks). For early disease (Langenskiold stage I-IV) bracing is the first line treatment, whereas stage V and VI patients normally require osteotomy.

29. **E** Talipes is associated with a range of congenital abnormalities including moulding disorders (e.g. high birth weight, DDH), soft tissue disorders (arthrogryposis) and dwarfisms. Males are more commonly affected than females. The features of Larsen's disease include hyper-mobility and multiple congenital subluxations/dislocations.

30. **D** SUFE is associated with obesity, male sex and thyroid disorders. It is diagnosed by a break in Klein's line (Trethowan's sign), widening of the capital epiphysis and increased head/neck angle. It is associated with a weakening of the perichondral ring and a fracture through the hypertrophic zone of the physis.

31. **D** Radial club hand is a common examination topic. It is a longitudinal deficiency of the forearm and may range from partial loss to complete absence of the radius, median nerve, radial artery and flexor carpi radialis. It is associated with TAR (thrombocytopaenia, absent radius syndrome), VACTERL (Vertebral abnormalities, Anal atresia, Cardiovascular anomlies, Tracheo-oEsophageal fistula, Renal and Limb defects), Fanconi's anaemia, and Holt-Oram syndrome (cardiac defects).

Extending Matching Answers

1. B   NICE guidance states that in the presence of a fragility fracture in the elderly, risk scoring or DEXA scan is not required, and if there are no contra-indications the patient should be started on bisphosphonate therapy.

2. A   There is no current screening programme for osteoporosis; as such, risk factor analysis such as FRAX is the first line in such patients before initiating any form of treatment.

3. D   The clinical vignette describes one of the contra-indications to bisphosphonate therapy. Bisphosphonates are known to cause osteonecrosis of the jaw, stress fractures of the femur and gastric ulcers. In a patient with severely depressed age-adjusted and raw BMD (T- and Z-scores respectively), an alternative therapy such as strontium should be initiated.

4. D   This patient has pseudoachondroplasia which is autosomal dominant (COMP gene mutation).

5. D   This patient has a congenital form of spondyloepiphyseal dysplasia, which is autosomal dominant (The *tarda* form is X-linked).

6. C   This patient has Gaucher's disease. Like all of the collagen storage diseases this is often associated with splenomegaly. Gaucher's is particularly associated with bilateral avascular necrosis of the hip.

7. A   This is the typical history for osteoid osteoma, which does not prolifically produce bone, but does directly activate the arachadonic acid pathway. This results in the typically strong analgesic effect of NSAIDs.

8. D   The history is typical for myositis ossificans. This typically ossifies from the outside in, whereas synovial cell carcinoma and other calcifying malignant soft tissue lesions tend to calcify from the inside out.

9. C   The patient has an enostosis or bone island. This is a benign asymptomatic area of mature bone seen within the metaphysis. An enostosis is cold on bone scan, and appears as a well circumscribed lesion demonstrating no periosteal reaction and a narrow zone of transition. There may be a coincidental history of trauma.

10. **E** Telangectatic osteosarcoma presents with lesions looking similar to aneurysmal bone cysts. However, the lesions are lytic, usually in the distal radius (often on the ulnar side). The doughnut sign (signifying central necrosis) and aggressive spread aid in differentiation from an ABC. In contrast to intramedullary osteosarcoma, the telangectatic form rarely demonstrates skip lesions and is less likely to present around the knee.

11. **B** The exact diagnosis in chondrosarcomas is partly based on the location of the lesion, as the histological and radiological characteristics can be difficult to differentiate. Chondrosarcoma presents in the 50+ age group, and responds poorly to both radiotherapy and chemotherapy.

Lesion	Characteristics
Intramedullary chondrosarcoma	Cartilage producing lesion with aggressive radiological and histological appearance. Seen in the pelvis and distal femur
Clear cell chondrosarcoma	Ephiphyseal location Large cells with central nuclei Commonly located in the proximal humerus and femur
Dedifferentiated chondrosarcoma	Very aggressive radiological appearance 50% present with pathological fracture

12. **A** Chondroblastoma is a malignant tumour of adolescence. Although seen in the epiphysis of the humerus and knee, it can commonly cross the physis.

13. **F** Bacterial seeding occurs to the small tortuous vessels that double back on themselves within the metaphysis of the growing long bone. This either establishes osteomyelitis (extra-articular physis) or septic arthritis (intra-articular physis e.g. hip, shoulder, elbow).

14.   D   A Salter-Harris type I fracture occurs exclusively through the physis. The hypertrophic zone (of maturation) is specifically injured as this is the weakest portion of the physis.

Salter-Harris	Location
I	Physis (zone of maturation)
II	Physis and metaphysis (Thurston-Holland fragment)
III	Physis and epiphyseal fragment (usually occurs to a partially fused physis)
IV	Through metaphysis and epiphysis
V	Crush to physis

15.   A   The groove of Ranvier is the entry point for differentiating mesenchymal stem cells. It may be damaged during crush injuries to the physis and has been implicated in growth arrest in high grade Salter-Harris fractures.

Chapter 11

Genetics and Growth

MCQ 20
EMQ 10

Multiple Choice Questions

1. What term describes the phenomenon whereby the number of chromosomes within a cell is not an exact multiple of the haploid set?
   a. Aneuploidy
   b. Chimaera
   c. Euploidy
   d. Polyploidy
   e. Mosaicism

2. What is the approximate age at which ossification of the pisiform takes place?
   a. 6 months
   b. 2 years
   c. 5 years
   d. 8 years
   e. 12 years

3. **Which zone within the physis is functionally least adversely affected by systemic physiological stresses?**

    a. Reserve zone
    b. Proliferative zone
    c. Maturation zone
    d. Hypertrophic zone
    e. Zone of provisional calcification

4. **Which of the following does NOT have a recognised association with radial hemimelia?**

    a. Thrombocytopaenia
    b. Atrial septal defect
    c. Tracheo-oesophageal fistula
    d. Hypoplasia of the adrenal zona glomerulosa
    e. Bilateral renal hypoplasia

5. **Mr. and Mrs. Bone both suffer from the little known disease Occult Recurrent Unvoluntary Kinesia (ORUK), although none of their parents had the condition. ORUK is known to follow normal Mendelian inheritance patterns. What is the probability that their first child will develop ORUK?**

    a. 0%
    b. 25%
    c. 33.3%
    d. 50%
    e. 100%

6. **Which one of the following statements regarding Down syndrome is FALSE?**

    a. Incidence is 1 per 650–800 live births
    b. Down patients have an increased risk of slipped upper femoral epiphysis
    c. 90% of cases arise due to non-dysjunction of chromosome 21 during the first meiotic division of oogenesis
    d. 30% of Down patients will die before the age of 45
    e. Only 20% of Down conceptions will result in a live birth

7. **Which one of the following statements regarding fibular hemimelia is TRUE?**

   a. It is less common than tibial hemimelia
   b. Estimated incidence is between 5–20 per million live births
   c. The left side is more commonly affected
   d. Coventry and Johnson have described five distinct types I–V
   e. Complete fibular hemimelia occurs less commonly than the incomplete form

8. **Which one of the following is NOT a recognised feature of Patau syndrome (trisomy 13)?**

   a. Post-axial polydactyly
   b. Microcephaly
   c. Microphthalmia
   d. Sacral agenesis
   e. Cleft palate

9. **Which one of the following statements regarding achondroplasia is TRUE?**

   a. Clinical features include rhizomelic micromelia
   b. Inheritance follows an autosomal recessive pattern
   c. Approximately 50% of cases occur as a result of a new mutation
   d. The defective gene is located on chromosome 5
   e. Patients classically have disproportionately short fibulae in relation to their tibiae

10. **Which one of the following conditions demonstrates an autosomal recessive inheritance pattern?**

    a. Duchenne muscular dystrophy
    b. Charcot-Marie-Tooth disease
    c. Holt-Oram syndrome
    d. Hypophosphataemic rickets
    e. Hurler's syndrome

11. **Which one of the following statements regarding meiosis is TRUE?**

    a. Two identical haploid gametes are produced from each cell entering the meiotic process
    b. Four identical haploid gametes are produced from each cell entering the meiotic process
    c. Crossing over between homologous chromosomes during prophase I significantly increases genetic diversity
    d. Prokaryotic cells can undergo meiotic division
    e. Meiosis occurs in the foetal central nervous system during the second trimester of pregnancy

12. **Which one of the following statements regarding the normal cell cycle is TRUE?**

    a. The majority of DNA synthesis occurs during the G_2 phase
    b. During the M phase, nuclear division (mitosis) is followed by division of the cell (cytokinesis)
    c. The G_1 phase leads directly into G_2
    d. Virtually all new DNA is synthesised during the G_0 phase
    e. Malignant cells spend a smaller proportion of the cell cycle in the G_0 phase

13. **In the physis, the hypertrophic zone:**

    a. Is the site at which slipping of the upper femoral epiphysis occurs in patients with renal failure
    b. Is the zone primarily affected in Morquio's syndrome
    c. Is the zone primarily affected in achondroplasia
    d. Has a high proteoglycan content
    e. Is a region of high oxygen tension

14. **Which of the lower limb physes is responsible for the greatest proportion of longitudinal growth?**

    a. Proximal femur
    b. Distal femur
    c. Proximal tibia
    d. Distal femur
    e. Proximal femur and distal tibia contribute roughly equally

15. **Which one of the following statements concerning foetal limb development is TRUE?**
    a. Mesenchymal differentiation and development occur under control from the apical ectodermal ridge
    b. The limb muscles derive innervation from dorsal rami of the spinal nerves
    c. During its development the lower limb undergoes 180° external rotation
    d. The upper limb buds start to form on approximately day 30 of gestation
    e. The development of secondary ossification centres is the precursor to formation of the elbow and knee joints

16. **The groove of Ranvier:**
    a. Firmly secures the epiphysis to the metaphysis
    b. Is contiguous peripherally with the metaphysis
    c. Is surrounded by the ring of Lacroix
    d. Is responsible for circumferential growth at the level of the epiphysis
    e. Is essential to the overall stability of the growth plate

17. **Which of the following is NOT a recognised feature of Turner's syndrome?**
    a. Cubitus valgus
    b. Medial tibial exostoses
    c. Shortening of 3rd metacarpal
    d. Scoliosis
    e. Osteoporosis

18. **Which of the following conditions is associated with the HLA-DR8 allele?**
    a. Addison's disease
    b. Reiter's syndrome
    c. Behçet's disease
    d. Pauciarticular juvenile rheumatoid arthritis
    e. Psoriatic arthritis

19. **Which one of the following processes does NOT involve endochondral ossification?**

    a. Development of primary ossification centre in the foetal limb
    b. Longitudinal long-bone growth
    c. Secondary fracture union
    d. Formation of the mandible
    e. Development of secondary ossification centre in epiphysis

20. **Which of the following conditions is caused by a defective gene on chromosome 17?**

    a. Neurofibromatosis type 1
    b. Christmas disease
    c. Hurler syndrome
    d. Achondroplasia
    e. Duchenne muscular dystrophy

Extended Matching Questions

SCENARIO I OPTIONS

A 11:22 chromosomal
   translocation
B X:18 chromosomal
   translocation
C Cartilage oligomeric matrix
   protein (COMP) gene
D COL 1A1 gene

E COL 1A2 gene
F Fibrillin gene
G FGF-receptor 3 gene
H RET gene
I PEX gene (cellular
   endopeptidase)
J SLC (sulphate or solute
   transporter) gene

For each of the following conditions, select the implicated gene or genetic mutation from the list above. Each option may be used once, more than once, or not at all.

1. Synovial sarcoma

2. Diastrophic dysplasia

3. Multiple endocrine neoplasia type I

4. Marfan syndrome

5. Ehlers-Danlos syndrome

SCENARIO II OPTIONS

A Epiphyseal hypoplasia   **E** Metaphyseal hypoplasia
B Epiphyseal hyperplasia   **F** Metaphyseal hyperplasia
C Physeal hypoplasia   **G** Diaphyseal hypoplasia
D Physeal hyperplasia   **H** Diaphyseal hyperplasia

For each of the following dysplasias, select the correct location and manifestation of the defect within the bone. Each option may be used once, more than once, or not at all.

6. Enchondromatosis

7. Craniometaphyseal dysplasia

8. Pseudoachondroplasia

9. Trevor's disease

10. Osteopetrosis

Answers: Chapter 11

MCQ 20
EMQ 10

Multiple Choice Answers

1. A The term ploidy refers to the number of sets of chromosomes in a biological cell. The haploid number is the number of chromosomes in a gamete. Any number of chromosomes that is not an exact multiple of the haploid number (human = 23) is termed *aneuploidy* – a well-known example is trisomy, where there are 47 chromosomes. Euploidy refers to the presence of 46 chromosomes (diploidy), polyploidy to an exact multiple greater than the diploid number – for example, triploidy (69 chromosomes). Chimaera refers to the presence of two different cell lines derived from two different zygotes. Mosaicism refers to different genetic cell lines that can be from multiple causes (e.g. meiosis errors), but both are derived from a single zygote.

2. E A knowledge of the rough age at which the different carpal bones ossify can be used to assess a child's age on the basis of wrist radiographs. This starts with the ulnar bones and progresses circumferentially, approximately as follows:

Capitate	6–12 months
Hamate	2 years
Triquetral	3 years
Lunate	4 years
Scaphoid	5 years
Trapezium	6 years
Trapezoid	6–7 years
Pisiform	12 years

3. E   The precise nomenclature of the different zones within the growth plate varies between texts; some include both maturation and calcification zones as 'sub-zones' within the hypertrophic zone. In any event, the phenomenon of Harris lines (transverse radiodense lines of calcification) is explicable by understanding that the zone of provisional calcification continues to function relatively normally at times when physiological stresses such as sepsis, trauma or malnutrition cause dysfunction of the zones closer to the physis. As a result, calcium deposition occurs without formation of new bone, resulting in a radiodense line.

4. D   Radial dysplasias, including hemimelia, have a number of recognised associations. Holt-Oram syndrome ('heart-hand syndrome') causes radial dysplasia and cardiac atrial septal defect; these may also occur as part of the wider VACTERL syndrome – Vertebral anomalies, Anal atresia, Cardiac abnormalities, Tracheo-Oesophageal fistula, Renal malformations (which may include bilateral hypoplasia), Limb abnormalities. Thrombocytopaenia may occur as part of the TAR syndrome (Thrombocytopaenia with Absent Radius). There is no known association with adrenal gland abnormalities.

5. E   The fact that none of the Bones' parents had ORUK, whilst they both developed the disorder, demonstrates that the inheritance pattern is autosomal recessive. However, the four parents must all have been carriers (i.e. assuming ORUK is expressed by the *o* allele whilst *N* is the normal allele, they would all have had *No* genotype). Mr. and Mrs. Bone both have *oo* genotype – if either carried the *N* allele they would not have expressed the ORUK phenotype. All of their children will therefore also express the ORUK phenotype as all will have the *oo* genotype. (ORUK of course really stands for Orthopeadic Research UK, not Occult Recurrent Unvoluntary Kinesia, which is not a genuine clinical entity!)

6. D   Trisomy 21 (Down syndrome) is the commonest trisomy, with estimated incidence 1 per 650–800 live births. Two thirds of conceptions will undergo spontaneous abortion during the first two trimesters, and of the remainder another third will fail to result in a live birth. Over 85% of live births will live into their 50s.

The vast majority result from a failure of dysjunction of chromosome 21 during the first meiotic division of oogenesis. Common orthopaedic manifestations include atlanto-axial subluxation, recurrent dislocations of the patella and an increased risk of slipped upper femoral epiphysis.

7. **B** Fibular hemimelia is the commonest of the long bone deficiency disorders, with an estimated incidence of 5.7–20 per million (*Florio et al, Fetal Diagn Ther* 1999). Most cases are unilateral, the right side is more commonly affected and the complete form is commoner than the incomplete form.

The Coventry and Johnson classification describes three types, with worsening prognosis:

Type I – partial unilateral fibular dysplasia; slight limb shortening may be the only sign

Type II – complete unilateral absence of fibula with associated tibial bowing, significant shortening and equinovalgus deformity of foot

Type III – cases presenting with type I or II deformities which are either bilateral, or are associated with other congenital abnormalities.

8. **D** The incidence of Patau syndrome is approximately 1 per 15000 live births; however, 6 month survivorship is 3% and those who do survive have severe mental and physical disability. Key clinical features include:

- Intrauterine growth retardation
- Cardiac abnormalities – septal defects, patent ductus arteriosus, dextrocardia
- Central nervous system – microcephaly, holoprosencephaly (failure of separation of two halves of forebrain), neural tube defects
- Craniofacial abnormailities – microphthalmia, scalp defects, cyclops, cleft lip and palate, deafness
- Limbs – post-axial polydactyly
- Abdominal – exomphalos, urogenital defects (polycystic kidneys, hypoplastic penis or clitoris)

Sacral agenesis has not been reported as a presenting feature.

9. A Achondroplasia affects approximately 1 in 10000 live births and is a form of disproportionate dwarfism i.e. the micromelia (limb shortening) demonstrates a rhizomelic morphology (the proximal part of the limb is disproportionately short), whilst the fibulae are disproportionately long relative to the tibiae. Although the condition follows an autosomal dominant inheritance pattern, almost 90% of cases result from new mutations. The defective FGF-receptor 3 (FGFR-3) gene is located on chromosome 4. Life expectancy and intelligence are unaffected.

10. E As a very broad general rule (albeit one with numerous exceptions), metabolic conditions are more likely to be recessive whilst structural ones have a tendency to be dominant. Hurler's mucopolysaccharidosis ('gargoylism') results from alpha-L iduronidase deficiency which leads to widespread accumulation of glycosaminoglycans (heparan sulphate and dermatan sulphate). Orthopaedic manifestations include widening of the medial clavicle, odontoid hypoplasia and progressive kyphosis due to anterior vertebral wedging. Death commonly occurs before the age of 10 due to cardio-respiratory complications.

Duchenne muscular dystrophy is an X-linked recessive disorder, whilst hypophosphataemic rickets is X-linked dominant. Charcot-Marie-Tooth and Holt-Oram are both autosomal dominant conditions.

11. C Meiosis is a process unique to eukaryotic organisms, allowing the generation of haploid gametes (spermatozoa or ova), which only takes place in the gonads (testes or ovaries). The process is broadly subdivided into meiosis I and II, each of which is further subdivided into prophase, metaphase, anaphase and telophase I and II respectively. During prophase I, crossing over occurs between homologous chromosomes, as a result of which new chromosomes are created containing a combination of maternal and paternal DNA – this significantly increases genetic variation. At the end of meiosis I two haploid daughter cells are produced; each of these undergoes further division (but this time with synthesis of new DNA) during meiosis II. In the male, the result is four non-identical haploid gametes; in the female only one gamete is produced, whilst the remaining cellular material is lost as the first and second polar bodies.

12. **B** The cell cycle is a sequence of steps involving the division of a cell and resulting in the formation of two further diploid cells. At any given time the majority of cells are in the quiescent G_0 phase, from where they may progress to one of two fates. The first is to undergo apoptosis (programmed cell death); the second is re-enter the active cell cycle to undergo division.

The active cell cycle is broadly divided into *interphase* (subdivided into G_1, S and G_2 phases) and the *M-phase*, comprising mitosis (nuclear division) and cytokinesis (cell division). During G_1, enzymes are produced that are used for intensive DNA synthesis in the S phase; from G_2 the cell leads directly into mitosis.

Malignancy occurs when the normal control mechanisms limiting cell division are lost. However, although within the total population the proportion of cells in the G_0 phase is reduced, the relative duration of each phase in not altered.

13. **B** In the hypertrophic zone, cells which have formed in the proliferative zone increase in size up to tenfold. This process is accompanied by a significant fall in both oxygen tension and proteoglycan concentration. This layer displays poor resistance to shear forces, and is therefore classically identified as the site through which growth plate injuries occur, including slipped upper femoral epiphysis (SUFE); an exception to this is seen in patients with renal failure, in whom SUFE more commonly occurs at the level of the primary spongiosa within the metaphysis. Hurler's and Morquio's mucopolysaccharidoses primarily affect the hypertrophic zone, whereas achondroplasia results from abnormal function within the proliferative zone.

14. **B** The majority of lower limb growth occurs around the knee (note that the opposite applies with regard to the upper limb and elbow – 'from the knee I flee, to the elbow I grow'). Additionally, the rate of growth in the distal femoral physis is approximately 50% higher than that in the proximal tibia.

15.   A The upper limb buds appear between days 24–26, the lower limb buds around day 28. Initially the limb buds comprise mesoderm with a basic overlying layer of ectodermal tissue; however, the zone of proliferating activity (ZPA) within the mesoderm secretes FGF-7 and -10 which leads to the development (and subsequent maintenance) of the apical ectodermal ridge (AER). The AER then has a central role as a control centre for activity in the underlying mesoderm; experimental evidence has shown that without the AER, limb development fails completely.

Synovial joint formation results from resorption and cavitation within mesenchyme that has undergone cartilaginous differentiation (the cartilage anlage) – the secondary ossification centres that develop at the ends of the long bones appear at a later stage. (Fibrous joints form directly as a result of differentiation of mesenchyme in fibrous tissue without cavitation taking place.)

During its development the lower limb undergoes 180° of internal rotation – this accounts for the dorsal flexion angle of the knee whilst that in the elbow is ventral. The skeletal muscles develop from myoblasts derived from the somites; this process starts proximally within the limb bud but distal migration rapidly occurs. Innervation is derived from the ventral rami.

16.   C The circumferential margin of the physis consists of 2 elements: the groove (or zone) of Ranvier and the perichondral ring of Lacroix. The groove of Ranvier is a wedge-shaped zone of chondrocytes, osteoblasts and fibroblasts which is contiguous peripherally with the epiphysis. The edge of the physis receives chondrocytes from the groove of Ranvier, which enables circumferential growth to occur at the level of the physis. The dense fibrous ring of Lacroix, which secures the epiphysis to the metaphysis and surrounds the zone of Ranvier, is a significant contributory factor to the overall stability of the growth plate.

17. C Turner's syndrome (monosomy of X-chromosome) affects 1 in 2000–2500 live female births (although 95% of Turner's foetuses spontaneously abort). Patients exhibit female phenotype, but with ovarian dysfunction and considerable shortening of stature (mean adult height is 20cm less than normal female average). Features include cubitus valgus, genu valgum, 4th (and sometimes 5th) metacarpal shortening, exostoses of the medial tibia, idiopathic scoliosis and webbing of the neck. There is a 5–10% incidence of coarctation of the aorta, and thyroid and other endocrine disorders are common. Osteoporosis is also a recognised feature, resulting from low plasma oestrogen levels.

18. D The HLA (or MHC) system is found on chromosome 6, and comprises a large number of genes encoding a variety of polypeptides, amongst which are numerous cell-surface antigen-presenting proteins. Some HLA associations worth memorising for the purposes of the exam are included below. However, some of these are under constant revision in the literature.

Condition	HLA- marker
Addison's disease	DR4
Ankylosing spondylitis	B27
Behçet's disease	B5, DR5, DQ2
Coeliac disease	DQ2, DQ8
Haemochromatosis	A3
Myasthenia gravis	DR3, DR6
Pauciarticular juvenile rheumatoid arthritis	DR5, DR8
Polyarticular juvenile rheumatoid arthritis	DR4, DR8
Psoriatic arthritis	B27
Reiter's syndrome	B27
Rheumatoid arthritis	DR1, DR4
Systemic lupus erythematosus	DR2, DR3
Sjögren's syndrome	B8, DR3

19. **D** Almost all bones are formed by endochondral ossification – the exceptions being the sternum, clavicles, flat bones of the skull and mandible. This is a process whereby cartilage is initially formed but then replaced by bone; the other form of ossification – intramembranous – occurring by the direct deposition of osteoid.

After the laying down of the cartilage model of the skeleton, primary ossification centres form in the cartilage within the central portion of the long bones. (At the same time, intramembranous ossification causes appositional growth to occur around the primary ossification centre.) The secondary ossification centres form later (the first, the distal femur, towards the end of gestation; the last, the clavicle, not until the third decade of life), but these too result from endochondral ossification. All longitudinal growth at the physis occurs via endochondral ossification, which is also responsible for secondary fracture union.

20. **A** NF-1 is caused by a mutation of the gene encoding neurofibromin, which is located on the long arm of chromosome 17. Some disease chromosomal locations that may be useful for exam purposes are included in the table below (note that many conditions, such as rheumatoid arthritis, are associated with genes found on more than one chromosome).

Condition	Chromosome
Achondroplasia	4
Ankylosing spondylitis	6
Charcot-Marie-Tooth disease	17
Christmas disease (haemophilia B)	X
Diastrophic dysplasia	5
Duchenne muscular dystrophy	X
Haemophilia A	X
Hurler's mucopolysaccharidosis	4
Marfan syndrome	15
Morquio's mucopolysaccharidosis	16
Neurofibromatosis I	17
Neurofibromatosis II	22
Osteogenesis imperfecta	17
Pseudoachondroplasia	19

Extending Matching Answers

1. B

2. J

3. H

4. F

5. E

Some of the commoner genetic associations encountered in orthopaedics are summarised as follows:

Disorder	Genetic association
Ewing's sarcoma	11:22 chromosomal translocation
Synovial sarcoma	X:18 chromosomal translocation
Rhabdomyosarcoma	2:13 chromosomal translocation
Myxoid lipsarcoma	12:16 chromosomal translocation
Chondrosarcoma	9:22 chromosomal translocation
Clear cell chondrosarcoma	12:22 chromosomal translocation
Multiple epiphyseal dysplasia	COMP gene
McCune-Albright syndrome	Gsα subunit gene
Osteogenesis imperfecta	COL 1A1, COL 1A2 genes
Schmid form of metaphyseal chondrodysplasia	COL 10A1 gene
Ehlers-Danlos Symdrome (certain subtypes)	COL 1A2 gene
Duchenne muscular dystrophy	Dystrophin gene (absent)
Becker muscular dystrophy	Dystrophin gene (abnormal)
Marfan syndrome	Fibrillin gene
Achondroplasia	FGF-receptor 3 gene
Neurofibromatosis I	Neurofibromin/NF1
Multiple Endocrine Neoplasia type I	RET gene
X-linked hypophosphataemic rickets	PEX gene (cellular endopeptidase)
Charcot-Marie-Tooth disease	PMP22 gene
Jansen metaphyseal chondrodysplasia	RTH-receptor P gene
Diastrophic dysplasia	Sulphate transporter gene

6. D

7. E

8. A

9. B

10. E

Rubin *(Arth Rheumatism 1964)* proposed a classification of bone dysplasias, still widely accepted, according to the level of the abnormality, along with whether cellular activity is hypo- or hyperplastic:

Rubin classification	Example conditions
Epiphyseal hypoplasia	Multiple epiphyseal dysplasia Spondyloepiphyseal dysplasia Pseudoachondroplasia
Epiphyseal hyperplasia	Dysplasia epiphysealis hemimelica (Trevor's disease)
Physeal hypoplasia	Achondroplasia Metaphyseal dysostosis
Physeal hyperplasia	Hyperchodroplasia Enchondromatosis
Metaphyseal hypoplasia	Osteopetrosis Craniometaphyseal dysplasia
Metaphyseal hyperplasia	Hereditary multiple exostoses
Diaphyseal hypoplasia	Osteogenesis imperfecta
Diaphyseal hyperplasia	Diaphyseal dysplasia

Chapter 12

Statistics and Data Interpretation

MCQ 25
EMQ 9

Multiple Choice Questions

1. Which of the following is a suitable measure of 'average' for non-parametric data?
   a. Mean
   b. Mode
   c. Median
   d. Standard deviation
   e. Interquartile range

2. Which of the following is the most suitable measure of spread about the mean?
   a. 95% confidence interval
   b. Standard error of the mean
   c. Mode
   d. Standard deviation
   e. Interquartile range

3. Which of the following distributions best describes the incidence of osteosarcoma in the UK population?
   a. Bi-modal
   b. Skewed
   c. Normal
   d. Excess kurtosis
   e. Parametric

4. **When applying Yates' correction to categorical data which of the following occurs?**

   a. Correction for the balinese paradox

   b. Correction for missed data points

   c. Conversion to non-parametric data

   d. Correction for small data sizes

   e. Binomial correction for sampling error

5. **The 'log-rank' test is usually used to demonstrate:**

   a. The significant difference between two calculated or observed curves

   b. The estimation of logistic regression constant for serial observations with multiple determinants

   c. Conversion of non-parametric to parametric data

   d. Estimation of difference in median between three non-parametric samples

   e. The correlation co-efficient for two sets of non-parametric data

6. **Which of the following is NOT a prerequisite when using the student's T-test?**

   a. Selection of 'number of tails'

   b. A positive D'Agostino omnibus normality test

   c. Parametric data

   d. A null hypothesis

   e. Continuous variables

7. **Which of the following statistical methods is appropriate for testing the significance of an observed difference in the number of ankle fractures united at the 12 week time point in a group of 3,000 smokers and non-smokers?**

   a. Fisher's exact test

   b. ANOVA

   c. ANOVA with a Bonferroni correction

   d. Mann-Whitney U-test

   e. Chi-squared test

8. **Which of the following statistical methods is appropriate for testing the significance of an observed difference in mean length to fracture union in ankle fractures between a group of 3,000 smokers and non-smokers?**

   a. Fisher's exact test
   b. Student's T-test
   c. Paired student's T-test
   d. Mann Whitney U-test
   e. Chi-squared test

9. **Which of the following statistical methods is appropriate for testing the significance of an observed difference in the number of ankle fractures united at 12 week and 16 week time points in a group of 3,000 smokers?**

   a. Fisher's exact test
   b. Student's T-test
   c. Paired student's T-test
   d. Mann Whitney U-test
   e. Chi-squared test

10. **Which of the following statistical methods is appropriate for testing the difference in a study with the results shown below?**

	Fracture healed	Fracture not healed
Non-smoker	51	7
Smoker	35	11

   a. Fisher's exact test
   b. Student's T-test
   c. Paired student's T-test
   d. Mann Whitney U-test
   e. Chi-squared test

11. Which of the following is the definition of sensitivity?

a. True positives/(true positives + false negatives)
b. True negatives/(true negatives + false positives)
c. True positives/(true positives + false positives)
d. True negatives/(true negatives + false negatives)
e. True positives/True negatives

12. Which of the following is the definition of positive predictive value?

a. True positives/(true positives + false negatives)
b. True negatives/(true negatives + false positives)
c. True positives/(true positives + false positives)
d. True negatives/(true negatives + false negatives)
e. True positives/True negatives

13. Which of the following statistical methods is suitable for analysis of significant difference between three or more non-parametric variables?

a. Pearson's test
b. Kruskal-Wallis
c. Paired two tailed T-test
d. Mann-Whitney U-test
e. Multiple logistic regression

14. **With regards to study design, which of the following definitions most closely describes a pragmatic randomised controlled trial?**
    a. Patients are recruited to a study and randomised to one treatment or another. Outcomes are assessed by an independent blinded observer and all management is controlled by trial protocol
    b. Patients are recruited to a study and randomised to one surgeon or another. Each surgeon carries out a different procedure. Outcomes are assessed by an independent blinded observer and all management is controlled by trial protocol
    c. Patients are recruited to a study and randomised to one treatment or another. Outcomes are assessed by the surgeon and all management is tailored to each patient
    d. Patients are recruited to a study and randomised to one treatment or another. Outcomes are assessed by an independent blinded observer and all management is tailored to individual patients
    e. Patients are recruited to allocate by 'block' in groups to one treatment or another. Outcomes are assessed by an independent blinded observer and all management is controlled by trial protocol

15. **Which of the following refers to the principle of analysing patient outcomes according to the initial management decision, even if they were unable to tolerate the intervention?**
    a. The primary outcome measure
    b. The secondary outcome measure
    c. Intention to treat analysis
    d. Biased based assessments
    e. None of the above

16. **Why is the concept of a 'null hypothesis' used in biostatistics?**

    a. A null hypothesis is a method for testing differences in studies which have no actual statistical purpose
    b. The 'null hypothesis' is not a biostatistics term and refers rather to an abstract mathematical concept
    c. The null hypothesis refers to a concept suggesting the opposite of the investigators' original thought is correct and is never formally statistically tested
    d. When determining what errors are associated with a study the construction of a null hypothesis allows for correction of potential observer bias
    e. It is statistically easier to disprove than prove a concept

17. **An investigator wishes to establish whether the age of patients is related to the reported pre-operative Oxford hip scores prior to undergoing total hip replacement. Which statistical method should she use?**

    a. Pearson's product moment correlation co-efficient
    b. Spearman's rank correlation co-efficient
    c. Chronbach's Alpha
    d. Co-efficient of variation
    e. Plot a scatter diagram

18. **With regards to meta-analyses, which of the following statements is FALSE?**

    a. Individual trials must be independently reviewed and assessed for bias
    b. It is permissible to contact authors to request additional data to assist in the production of summated result
    c. Forest plots may be used to depict evidence weight and outcome from individual trials and summed data
    d. Studies conforming to the CONSORT guidelines should be included in any meta-analysis on the subject
    e. Meta-analysis yields 'level one evidence' data and is the gold standard against which all other evidence must be measured

19. **With regards to systematic review, which of the following statements is FALSE?**

    a. Level V evidence should not be included in systematic reviews as it represents opinion only
    b. The Cochrane collaboration do not publish systematic reviews
    c. Thorough literature searches using recognised medical search engines with the search method should be clearly described in the methodology
    d. No statistical analysis is required
    e. The authors may state their personal opinion on the subject without the support of referenced or included studies

20. **Which of the following statements regarding statistical confidence intervals is TRUE?**

    a. The calculated 95% confidence interval for Kaplan-Meier survivorship analysis is independent of the sample size
    b. Where confidence intervals between two observed means do not overlap the two study populations are always statistically significantly different
    c. In interval analysis of two population means, the confidence intervals for subsequent observations will continue to widen, assuming the study population size remains the same and there is a constant loss to follow-up rate
    d. Confidence interval is calculated in a variety of different manners but in all cases is related to the standard error of the mean and the results of a significance test (T-test)
    e. When constructing a life table analysis, confidence intervals are irrelevant when comparing survivorship for two different cohorts as the life tables method does not require confidence intervals to be reported

21. Which of the following statements regarding averages is FALSE?

a. The mean is a method of analysing 'average' which is defined as the sum of all values divided by the number of values. It is suitable for parametric data

b. The median is a method of analysing 'average' which may be used for ordinal as well as continuous data. It is often used to estimate average in non-parametric data

c. The standard error of the mean is a method of estimating the accuracy of which the study mean represents the population mean. It is sensitive to the study size, distribution of values and range of observed values

d. In normally distributed data the median and mean will give the same value

e. The mode refers to the most frequent observation – and would, for example, be an appropriate analysis method for a study investigating the most common population height

22. Which of the following statements regarding logistic regression analysis is FALSE?

a. Multiple logistic regression analysis can be used to estimate the contribution of multiple variables to a known dichotomous outcome

b. Logistic regression analysis may only be used for a single type of data (i.e. it is not possible to mix ordinal and continuous data within the same analysis)

c. Simple linear regression analysis assumes that a continuous outcome variable can be defined as $y = (c_0 + c_1) * (x_1 + C_2) * (x_2 + c_3) \ldots$ etc.

d. It is possible to utilise logistic regression to produce p values to assess the significance of a variable as a determinant of continuous outcome variables

e. Multiple logistic regression can be used with an interaction model to assess interdependence of variables

23. **The CONSORT statement is a consensus statement about the design of randomised controlled trials (RCTs). Which one of the following is FALSE?**

    a. The CONSORT statement recommends the 'ideal standard' for reporting randomised trials. A well conducted study may not fulfil all of the criteria but should fulfil over 20 of the 25 item check list

    b. The CONSORT statement recognises the occasional need to change trial design after the commencement of the trial

    c. The CONSORT statement recognises the need to register RCTs and to have freely available trial protocols

    d. The CONSORT statement requires determination of the study size by a recognised statistical method before the trial begins

    e. It is possible not to blind patients or investigators in a randomised controlled trial and still fulfil the CONSORT guidance

24. **A group wishes to design a study to examine patients' feelings of depression, and the causes of this, following major injury. Which one of the following would be the most appropriate study design?**

    a. A qualitative research study beginning with prospective recruitment; patient scoring with depressive indexes and pairwise multiple significance testing could then be assessed using t-testing coupled with root cause analysis methods

    b. A quantitative research study based around allocation of patients into injury type and depressive level, with subsequent Kruskal-Wallis tests

    c. A qualitative analysis using patient focus groups and recorded patient interviews, but without any formal statistical testing

    d. A quantitative analysis using depressive indicies linked to length of stay and 'depressive triggers'

    e. Observational commentary through patient diaries and independent monitors to assess mood at specific trigger points

25. **When performing a power analysis it is usual to power a study for:**

   a. Alpha error 0.05, Beta error 0.01
   b. Alpha error 0.95, Beta error 0.05
   c. Alpha error 0.05, Beta error 0.95
   d. Alpha error 0.05, Beta error 0.80
   e. Alpha error 0.80, Beta error 0.05

Extended Matching Questions

SCENARIO I OPTIONS

A Patients are recruited to a pilot screening programme for osteoporosis by leaflet at 'well woman check' health screening clinics at 10 GP practices. The screening programme is deemed a failure as only 2% of the 3,000 women recruited have osteoporosis.

B A practice nurse conducts a prospective study investigating the attitudes of patients towards health care advice. She places a poster advertising the study in the waiting room. It is a qualitative study performed by covertly recording patient consultations and then analysing the conversation for themes.

C A surgeon conducts a randomised trial of minimal vs traditional total hip replacement. He reviews all the patients in clinic himself and administers a Harris Hip Score after scoring the wound healing.

D An FY2 doctor, as part of the departmental audit, sends some questionnaires to patients. A patient complains to the trust PALS service.

E An investigator wishes to establish the causative factors of death after surgery for fractured neck of femur. He investigates 37 factors and finds one (sex) to be significant with a p value of 0.05.

F A prospective comparative cohort series is undertaken to investigate the potential benefit of double bundle ACL reconstruction over single bundle. The study includes 25 patients in each arm after power analysis shows 24 are required. Five patients drop out and no difference in found in functional scores.

G Two nurses and a physio each administer the same clinician reported outcome tool to the same group of five patients to assess its reliability.

This question relates to faults with clinical study design. For each of the faults described, choose from the list of scenarios the example which most accurately reflects the error in question.

1. The study may suffer from a Type 1 error.

2. The study suffers from a Type 2 error.

3. The study suffers from selection bias.

SCENARIO II OPTIONS

A Parametric data   E Nominal data
B Non-parametric data   F Qualitative data
C Ordinal data   G Skewed data
D Categorical data

For each of the following study descriptions, select from the options above the type of data most likely to be generated. Each option may be used once, more than once, or not at all.

4. A comparative study is performed in patients undergoing surgical treatment of a femoral fracture, to assess the correlation between the patient's forearm length and the diameter of femoral nail inserted. The primary outcome measure is in millimetres and Pearson's test is performed.

5. A consultant follows up all of his total hip arthroplasty patients and scores them with the Harris hip score, and reports the results according to the original outcomes described, as Excellent, Good, Fair or Poor.

6. A GP conducts a series of interviews with patients to investigate their experience when using the outpatient gynaecology service offered by his practice. He investigates the women's perceptions of the positive aspects of the GP-led service thoroughly, using structured interviews.

SCENARIO III OPTIONS

A Level 1   **E** Case-matching
B Level 2   **F** Case-controlled
C Level 3   **G** Case series
D Level 4

This question concerns levels of evidence. For each of the following study scenarios, select the correct level of evidence from the list above. Each option may be used once, more than once, or not at all.

7. The investigator compares the results of patients undergoing a new treatment to the outcomes from a group of previous patients having a different intervention. The second (previous) intervention group are carefully selected such the groups as closely as possible match each other.

8. A study is constructed and patients are randomised between two different knee interventions; arthroscopy and washout, or arthroscopy and debridement of degenerate meniscal tears. Due to the consent process, however, patients were inadvertently made aware of the intervention they were receiving.

9. The national joint registry is a population study of every patient receiving a total joint arthroplasty.

Answers: Chapter 12

MCQ 25
EMQ 9

Multiple Choice Answers

1. C Median is the most suitable measure of 'average' for non-parametric data as all other measures are subject to skew by the non-parametric nature of the data. Mode is most useful in ordinal measures and mean for parametric data.

2. D Mean is the most suitable measure of parametric data, which is either normally distributed or has been transformed to a normal distribution. Standard deviation is the measure of spread about the mean, with 90% of values falling within one standard deviation and 95% within two. Interquartile range is the appropriate measure of spread for non-parametric data. 95% confidence intervals and standard error of the mean are measures of accuracy of estimation of the mean.

3. A Bi-modal distribution describes data spread with two peaks in incidence, such as osteosarcoma with primary occurring earlier than the later secondary osteosarcomas. Other distribution types described are:

Skewed – Where there is higher propensity for an observation to lie to one side of the geometric mean than the other

Normal – The classic bell-shaped distribution. 95% of data lie within 2 standard deviations and 97.5% within 3 SDs of the mean.

Kurtosis is a measure of skew and parametric data occur when the data can be described by, or transformed to a parabolic curve, normally a bell curve.

4. D Yates's correction is a *post-hoc* (after significance testing) correction for the Chi squared test that can be used to account for small numbers within categorical data.

5. A The log-rank test is used to test the significant difference between two curves, either calculated or otherwise. In orthopaedics it is often used for testing the difference between two survivorship curves.

6. B The D'Agostino omnibus normality test aims to establish whether a sample comes from a normally distributed population. Whilst parametric data is required for a student's T-test there is no requirement to perform formal normality testing. Data must be transformed to a normal distribution or corrections made for skew. All the other conditions listed are requirements.

7. E Categorical data such as this (yes/no answers resulting in percentages) must be analysed with contingency table analysis. Significance testing is then undertaken with either a Chi-squared or Fisher's exact test. Fisher's modification to the Chi-squared test is only suitable for small sample sizes; hence Chi-squared is the correct answer here.

The Mann-Whitney is suitable for analysis of non-parametric data and the ANOVA a complex group of analyses which address multiple (more than two) groups, abnormal or uneven distributions and can also be corrected for multiple testing errors.

8. B This question concerns parametric data from two different groups which is likely to have a normal distribution. This is best tested with a student's T-test. The Mann-Whitney U-test is used for non-parametric continuous data.

9. C Multiple observations at two different time points are best analysed using a paired student's T-test which is the only listed test suitable for multiple different observations. Other suitable tests for multiple testing include a two-way ANOVA or mANOVA tests.

10. A Due to the small number of samples in the 'non-smoker/not healed' group a Fisher's exact test is suitable to analyse the data. Fisher's exact test is in general indicated when there are fewer than 10 observations in any cell of a contingency table.

11. A Sensitivity refers to the proportion of patients who have a condition who test positive. Response B relates to specificity, or the proportion of patients testing negative who really do not have the condition.

12. C The positive predictive value (PPV or precision rate) quantifies the number of patients with a positive result who in fact have the condition being tested for. Conversely the negative predictive value, given by equation D, refers to the proportion of those testing negative who genuinely do not have the condition.

13. B The Kruskal-Wallis one way analysis of variance is suitable for non-parametric multiple significance testing. Logistic regression is used to determine the proportion of effect of an individual variable in determining (or predicting) outcomes.

Pearson's test is used for parametric correlations (Spearman's for non-parametric correlation). The tails on a T-test refer to the acceptable number of assumptions. Single tailed T-tests should not be used unless it is clear the opposite of the observed difference could never occur under any circumstance.

14. D With a pragmatic trial design the important elements of the study are controlled, but less important elements are not – for example post-operative follow-up regimen or subsequent investigations. Answer A describes a randomised blinded controlled trial; B blinded randomisation to treatment package; C a randomised trial; E a comparative blinded case series.

15. C In randomised controlled trials patients are reported on an intention to treat basis according to the allotted treatment group, irrespective of the outcome.

16. E It is exceedingly difficult to prove statistically that there is a difference between observations, and much easier to prove there is 'not no difference'; hence the 'null hypothesis' is used for ease of computation, which once disproved, proves the hypothesis.

17. A Age and the Oxford hip score both approximate to parametric data and have a Gaussian distribution. This association can be quantified by the Pearson's correlation co-efficient. Spearman's test is for non-parametric data, Chronbach's Alpha for levels of agreement.

18. E Meta-analysis is a data synthesis method. The level of evidence of a meta-analysis depends on the studies included. If rigorous statistical methods are not adhered too and Level II and below data included then the meta-analysis itself is level II evidence. All of the other points are true. CONSORT is a consensus statement for well conducted randomised controlled trials.

19. A Systematic reviews are articles synthesising the current literature. They may include all levels of evidence including the personal opinions of the authors and all levels of evidence.

20. C Confidence intervals are the estimation of the accuracy to which the mean of the sample population reflects the mean of the general population. They are essential in all types of analysis; if there is an on-going loss to follow-up the confidence intervals will continue to widen.

21. E Although the mode does refer to the most frequent observation it is not suitable for analysis of a continuous variable like population height, only for ordinal and categorical data analysis.

22. D Logistic regression is only suitable for dichotomous end points so answer D is incorrect.

23. A The CONSORT statement is a minimum reporting standard, not an ideal standard. The CONSORT statement is equally applicable to less robust study designs such as alteration to trial design, interim analysis and non-blinded trials.

24. C Qualitative analysis is required using standard methodology as described. There are quantitative analysis methods that can be used for exploratory psychological studies like this one. Answer E is a time and motion observational study and will not assess cause.

25. D Although these values are arbitrary, it is commonly accepted that alpha (type 1) error should be set at 5% and beta (type 2) error at 80% in most biological studies. Type 1 error refers to the incorrect rejection of a true null hypothesis; in type 2 error, a false null hypothesis is wrongly accepted.

Extending Matching Answers

1. E It would be expected by random chance that one in 20 significance tests would be positive if p=0.05. Therefore this study is at risk of a type 1 error due to multiple pairwise analysis.

2. F Although the investigators have conducted a power analysis, their study has become underpowered due to four patients having dropped out; therefore the lack of significant difference may be due to a type 2 error.

3. A This study suffers from selection bias (albeit unintentional) as the patients are already seeking healthcare advice, and so are less at risk of osteoporosis than the general population.

4. A Lengths are normally distributed and are continuous. Pearson's test is the correct test to correlate parametric data.

5. C The data are ordinal (ordered data) as the outcomes are in order, but still discrete data.

6. F Patient experience research is nearly always qualitative.

7. E This is an example of case matching. A case controlled study investigates a group of patients receiving the same intervention.

8. B This is a poorly constructed RCT, so constitutes level 2 evidence.

9. A This is not a case series as every patient in the country is added on to the register, making it a level 1 population study.

Chapter 13

Hand and Wrist

MCQ 16
EMQ 9

Multiple Choice Questions

1. Which is the most important pulley in the thumb?
   a. A1 pulley
   b. A2 pulley
   c. Oblique pulley
   d. C1 pulley
   e. C2 pulley

2. A 58-year-old lady with rheumatoid arthritis presents with an inability to extend her ring and little finger. Which of the following could be the cause?
   a. Extensor tendon rupture
   b. Trigger finger
   c. Metacarpophalangeal joint subluxation
   d. Posterior interosseous nerve palsy
   e. All of the above

3. After repair of flexor digitorum profundis to the middle finger a patient notices that while trying to make a fist only the middle finger reaches the palm. The name for this phenomenon is:
   a. Rugger jersey finger
   b. Mallet finger
   c. Boutonniere deformity
   d. Quadrigia
   e. Lumbrical plus deformity

4. **Limited passive flexion of PIP when the MCPJ is extended but normal passive flexion of the PIPJ when the MCPJ is flexed is caused by:**

   a. Extensor tendon adhesions
   b. Intrinsic muscle contracture
   c. Lumbrical minus finger
   d. Capsular tightness
   e. Flexor tendon adhesions

5. **What is the largest contributing factor to the strength of a flexor tendon repair?**

   a. Diameter of suture crossing the repair
   b. Number of strands crossing the repair
   c. The presence of an epitendinous suture
   d. The use of a non-absorbable suture material
   e. The presence of braiding in the suture

6. **The so called DISI (dorsal intercalated segment instability) deformity of the wrist is a result of an injury to which ligament?**

   a. Scapholunate ligament
   b. Triangular ligament
   c. Lunotriquetral
   d. Dorsal radiotriquetral
   e. Volar radioscapholunate ligament

7. **Which of the following ligaments need to be injured to cause a VISI (volar intercalated segment instability) deformity?**

   a. Lunotriquetral and dorsal radiotriquetral
   b. Lunotriquetral and scapholunate
   c. Dorsal radiotriquetral and scapholunate
   d. Dorsal radiotriquetral and volar radioscaphoid
   e. Lunotriquetral and radioscapholunate

8. **Which of the following is NOT a component of the TFCC?**
   a. Origin of ulnolunate ligament
   b. Origin of lunotriquetral ligament
   c. Articular disc
   d. Volar radioulnar ligament
   e. Tendon sheath of FCU

9. **A 60-year-old man sustained a distal radius fracture that was treated non-operatively three months ago. He now presents with a sudden inability to extend his thumb. What is the likely aetiology?**
   a. EPL rupture
   b. EPB rupture
   c. FPL entrapment
   d. Sagittal band disruption
   e. Lateral band subluxation

10. **Which one of the following anatomical structures in the hand is unaffected by Dupuytren's disease?**
    a. Natatory ligament
    b. Grayson's ligament
    c. Cleland's ligament
    d. Spiral band
    e. Lateral digital sheet

11. **Which one of the following cells is found in the early stages of Dupuytren's disease?**
    a. Fibroblast
    b. Myofibroblast
    c. Macrophage
    d. Giant cell
    e. CD 8+ leucocyte

12. **A complete laceration to the ulnar nerve at the elbow causes which characteristic hand deformity?**
    a. DIP extension of little and ring
    b. MCPJ hyperextension and flexion of little and ring IPJs
    c. MCPJ flexion and hyperextension of little and ring IPJs
    d. Hyperextension of index and middle at MCPJs
    e. PIPJ flexion

13. **Pacinian corpuscles respond to which kind of stimulus?**
    a. Pressure
    b. Joint position
    c. Temperature
    d. Pain
    e. Light touch

14. **An injury to the volar plate of the PIPJ of the middle finger can progress to:**
    a. A mallet deformity
    b. A swan neck deformity
    c. A rugger jersey deformity
    d. A boutonniere deformity
    e. A Z deformity

15. **Which of the following muscles should not be sacrificed for use as a donor tendon in transfer to correct a peripheral nerve lesion?**
    a. Extensor carpi radialis brevis and extensor carpi radialis longus
    b. Extensor carpi radialis brevis and abductor pollicis longus
    c. Brachioradialis and palmaris longus
    d. Extensor indicis and extensor carpi radialis brevis
    e. Pronator teres and flexor carpi radialis

16. A 60-year-old man sustained a distal radius fracture that was treated operatively six months ago with a volar locking plate. He now presents with difficulty holding a pen. What is the likely aetiology?

    a. EPL rupture
    b. EPB rupture
    c. FPL rupture
    d. Sagittal band disruption
    e. Lateral band subluxation

Extended Matching Questions

SCENARIO I OPTIONS

A Intrinsic plus hand
B Intrinsic minus hand
C Boutonniere deformity
D Capsular tightness
E Lumbrical plus finger
F Swan neck deformity

G Central slip dysfunction
H Mallet deformity
I Sagittal bands
J Oblique retinacular ligament
K Scapholunate ligament
L Intersection syndrome

Which of the responses above best fit each of the following definitions? Each option may be used once, more than once or not at all.

1. Which pathological process leads to a flexion deformity of the PIP and an extension deformity of the DIP?

2. An untreated disruption of the terminal extensor mechanism can lead to this deformity.

3. Combined low median and ulnar nerve injury can lead to this deformity.

4. Which structure is injured in the little finger of a boxer with extensor tendon subluxation?

5. A patient presents with difficulty flexing the finger at the PIPJ. An examiner finds that there is equally reduced excursion of the PIPJ with the MCPJ flexed or extended.

6. Which pathological process leads to difficulty passively flexing the DIPJ when the PIPJ is extended?

7. Whilst radially deviating the wrist, a dorsally directed pressure is applied to the volar surface of the wrist; there is a clunk as the pressure is removed. Which structure is affected?

8. While attempting to grip a beer glass the history student complains of his middle finger extending. He vaguely remembers hurting this finger while playing rugby 6 months ago.

9. A 22-year-old college oarsman complains of radial-sided wrist pain after increasing training

Answers: Chapter 13

> MCQ 16
> EMQ 9

Multiple Choice Answers

1. C In the thumb there are only two annular pulleys and one oblique pulley. The A1 pulley overlies the MCP joint, the A2 overlies the IP joint and the oblique pulley lies inbetween, overlying the shaft of the proximal phalanx. The oblique pulley is the most important.

2. E The question is deliberately vague about the history. All of the above are possible causes (as is ulnar subluxation of extensor tendons). Clinical examination is necessary to differentiate the causes.

3. D The quadrigia effect occurs because FDP is a multipennate muscle. Shortening one of the tendons will result in that finger 'bottoming out' in the palm before the others have fully closed, thus presenting as the inability to make a fist. In this case the cause would be a surgical shortening of the FDP during operative repair.

4. B The stem describes a positive Bunnell test for intrinsic muscle contracture. This clinical presentation is caused by an imbalance between tight intrinsic muscles (interossei and lumbricals). At rest the hand assumes a posture of MCPJ flexion and both DIPJ and PIPJ extension.

The Bunnell test differentiates between the intrinsic and extrinsic tightness. Firstly the passive movement of the finger joints should be checked to make sure that they are normal. Then the test involves passive flexion of the PIPJ when the MPJ is either flexed or extended. The test is positive if there is less PIP flexion when the MCPJ is extended than when it is flexed. This arises because the MCP extension stretches the intrinsic muscles. The stretch on the already shortened intrinsic muscles leads to an extensor force on the IPJs which prevents flexion. Restricted PIPJ flexion when the MCPJ is in both fixed and extended positions implicates another cause, like capsular tightness, whereas restricted PIPJ flexion only with the MCPJ extended implicates intrinsic tightness.

5. B The number of strands of core suture crossing the repair is the principle contributor to repair strength with up to eight core suture strands recommended, a locking suture with the knot away from the repair site, a good purchase of suture, and an epitendinous suture.

Other factors deemed important in the strength of the repair are the use of non-absorbable suture, dorsal as opposed to volar placement of the suture, and better purchase of the core suture.

6. A See answer to question 7.

7. A The DISI and VISI deformities are categorised by the position/inclination of the lunate on the lateral radiograph. To be classified as a DISI deformity the lunate has to be extended, with the degree of extension necessary to be classified as a DISI being a scapholunate angle of >60 degrees (normal 47, range 30–60). The causes, amongst others, include SLL tear and scaphoid fracture.

Conversely to be classified as a VISI deformity the scapholunate angle has to be < 30 degrees. It is caused by disruption of the lunotriquetral ligament and dorsal radiotriquetral ligament.

The radioscapholunate ligament is the ligament of Testut – it is a vascular conduit and not a true ligament.

8. E The TFCC is made up of the following structures:

- Ulnolunate and lunotriquetral (ulnocarpal) ligaments
- Dorsal and volar radioulnar ligament
- Articular disc
- Meniscal homologue
- Ulnar collateral ligament
- ECU subsheath

9. A EPL rupture can occur after operatively or conservatively treated distal radius fractures. The incidence may be as high as 5% in conservatively treated fractures. The aetiology is thought to be an attrition of the tendon secondary to its impingement upon a healing callus or a pressure effect of haematoma in the EPL sheath.

Roth K., Incidence of Extensor Pollicis Longus Tendon Rupture After Non-displaced Distal Radius Fractures. J Hand Surg 2012 May 37(5), 942–7

10. C In Dupuytren's disease the normal anatomical fascial bands become diseased and are renamed "cords" (bands make cords). The common cords are:

- central (in continuity with pretendinous cord)
- lateral (a diseased lateral digital sheath)
- abductor digiti minimi
- natatory cords.

The spiral cord is composed of:

- pretendinous band
- spiral band
- lateral digital sheath
- Grayson's ligament.

All four of these structures spiral around the neurovascular bundle. The neurovascular bundle is brought in the palmar direction, proximally and towards the midline. Cleland's ligament is not involved in the disease process.

11. B Dupuytren's disease is staged by Luck into proliferative, involutional and residual stages. The cell type seen in stages 1 and 2 is the myofibroblast. With progression though the stages there is a dense myofibrinous network and a large amount of type III collagen, leading to a high type III to type I ratio. In the residual stage the myofibroblasts disappear to leave the fibrocytes as the predominant cell type.

12. B Division of the ulnar nerve at the wrist paralyses all of the small muscles of the hand except the first and second lumbricals, opponens pollicis, abductor pollicis brevis and flexor pollicis brevis. The clinical presentation is hyperextension of the 4th and 5th fingers at the MCP joints and flexion at the IPJs. With more proximal lesions of the ulnar nerve this posture is less severe because the long flexors producing the IPJ flexion are also denervated – the so called "ulnar paradox".

13. A The end sensory organs in the skin are:

- Pacinian corpuscle
    - *vibration and pressure*
- Meissner corpuscle
    - *light touch – rapidly adapting*
- Merkel receptor
    - *sustained touch and pressure*
- Ruffini corpuscle
    - *skin stretch*

14. B The swan neck deformity is characterised by hyperextension of the PIPJ with flexion of the DIPJ. The deformity can begin at PIPJ or DIPJ (or even MCPJ). See EMQ 2 for the underlying anatomical changes.

Causes:

MCPJ: Intrinsic tightness – MCPJ subluxation and PIP hyperextension

PIPJ: Hyperextension due volar plate laxity

FDS: Rupture

DIPJ: Mallet deformity

Loss / dysfunction of central slip

Other causes are generalised inflammatory joint disease, such as rheumatoid arthritis, causing a mixture of the above pathologies.

15. A There are no absolute contra-indications to any particular tendon transfers. Some sources recommend never sacrificing extensor carpi radialis brevis but a combination of ECRB and ECRL should not be sacrificed together as without them wrist extension cannot be easily achieved. (See also Chapter 4, MCQ 19)

Dell, P. Ulnar Intrinsic Anatomy and Dysfunction J Hand Ther. 2005;18:198–207.

16. C FPL rupture is associated with the use of volar locking plates. This can occur chronically and is probably an attrition rupture of FPL.

Extending Matching Answers

1. G This question describes a boutonniere deformity. The mechanism underlying this deformity is dysfunction of the central extensor slip (inserting into the base of the middle phalanx). Weakening or disruption of the central slip leads to loss of active PIPJ extension and with the unbalanced extensor mechanism the FDS forces a continued flexion of the PIPJ. Subsequent attenuation of the triangular ligament results in migration of the lateral bands volarly. Here they can only act to flex the PIPJ and hyperextend the DIPJ.

2. F Untreated mallet deformity can lead to a swan neck deformity of the PIPJ due to an imbalance of the extensor mechanism. Laxity of the transverse retinacular ligament results in subluxation of the conjoined lateral band to lie dorsal to the axis of rotation of the PIPJ. Secondary shortening of the transverse ligament maintains it there. The dorsal placement of the lateral band leads to hyperextension of the PIPJ and loss of extension of the DIPJ. Secondary processes include laxity of the PIPJ volar plate, intrinsic muscle tightness and collateral ligament contracture.

3. B The intrinsic minus hand is a claw hand with hyperextension of MCP joints and flexion of the PIP and DIP joints. The deformity is produced by an imbalance of the intrinsics and extrinsics. The intrinsic muscles are weakened or paralysed such that the normal long extensor muscles, unopposed, hyperextend the MCP joint, and the long flexor muscles flex the PIP and DIP joints.

Causes, amongst others are combined low median and ulnar nerve lesion and brachial plexus injuries. They will give different patterns of clawing depending upon the nerve(s) involved.

4. I The sagittal bands anchor the extensor tendon over the central MCP joint. Injury of the sagittal bands most often involves tear of the sagittal hood on the radial side of finger following trauma, classically in boxing. Severe tears result in subluxation into the gully between the metacarpals and the patient will be unable actively to extend the finger from a flexed position. However, if the finger is passively extended (and the tendon thus relocated); the patient will be able to keep the finger extended.

5. D The question describes Bunnell's test, which aims to distinguish intrinsic tightness from other causes of joint contracture e.g. capsular tightness. Flexion of the PIPJ is tested with the MCPJ either flexed or extended. The test is positive if there is less PIP flexion when the MCPJ is extended than when it is flexed. A negative test implies another cause e.g. capsular tightness.

6. J The described condition is caused by tightness of the Oblique Retinacular Ligament (ORL). The ORL runs from flexor tendon sheath on the volar surface of the finger at the proximal phalanx to the terminal extensor tendon (on the dorsum of the finger). It serves to link the motion of DIP and PIP joints. Flexion of the PIP joint results in relaxation of the ORL, thereby allowing DIP flexion. Conversely, extension of the PIPJ tightens the ORL which in turn assists DIP extension.

The test for ORL tightness involves holding the PIPJ in extension while passively flexing the DIPJ. If the ORL is tight it is not possible passively to flex the DIPJ. However, when the PIPJ is passively flexed then passive flexion of the DIPJ is possible.

7. K This is the Kirk Watson test, in which the hand is placed in ulnar deviation and an examiner presses on the proximal pole of the scaphoid from the volar to dorsal direction. The wrist is then moved from ulnar to radial deviation. If the SLL is incompetent then normal flexion of the scaphoid is not possible and the dorsally directed pressure drives the scaphoid off the dorsal rim of the radius. Upon releasing the dorsally directed pressure the scaphoid relocates with a clunk – a positive test.

8. E This describes a lumbrical plus finger. Each lumbrical arises from the FDP tendon and inserts onto the radial sided lateral band of each finger. If the FDP has been disrupted distal to the origin of the lumbrical then it will shorten. If the FDP then contracts while trying to grip an object the lumbrical is tightened and pulls on the lateral band, which in turn causes PIPJ and DIPJ extension. This gives rise to the paradoxical extension of the IPJs while attempting to flex the fingers.

9. L From the options available this presentation describes intersection syndrome. It is due to inflammation of the tendons as the first dorsal wrist compartment (EPB and APL) crosses over the second compartment (ECRL and ECRB). It is common in rowers and weight lifters (and can occur in golfers who are changing their swing). There is pain and often crepitus over the dorsoradial forearm and pain with resisted wrist dorsiflexion and radial deviation.

Chapter 14

Biomechanics

MCQ 40
EMQ 17

Multiple Choice Questions

1. **In the shoulder, the position of 90° of forward flexion, 15° of adduction and maximum internal rotation is reported to stress which structure?**
   a. Superior labrum
   b. Inferior glenohumeral ligament
   c. Inferior labrum
   d. Posterior labrum
   e. Middle glenohumeral ligament

2. **Which of the following measurements about the orientation of the shoulder joint is INCORRECT?**
   a. The humeral articular surface is retroverted 30° with respect to the condylar axis of the humerus
   b. The glenoid is tilted upwards about 5°
   c. The glenoid is anteverted about 7°
   d. The scapular plane is between 30° to 50° anterior to the coronal plane of the body
   e. During abduction of the arm there is a 2:1 ratio of glenohumeral:scapulothoracic motion

3. **Which of the following best describes the functional anatomy and movement at the glenohumeral joint?**
   a. The centre of rotation of the shoulder moves significantly from the centre of the glenoid during shoulder movement
   b. Anterior ligaments are tight in internal rotation
   c. A deficiency of the anterosuperior labrum in association with a cord-like MGHL is a normal anatomical variant
   d. Deltoid is less effective with increasing elevation of the arm
   e. Abduction is initiated by deltoid

4. **Which of the following best describes movement at the elbow joint?**
   a. Movement is possible in five degrees of freedom
   b. The rotational axis for flexion-extension is through the centre of the capitellum
   c. The anterior oblique ligament of the medial collateral ligament is taut throughout flexion and extension
   d. The most important stabiliser to varus stress is the lateral collateral ligament
   e. Full range of movement of the elbow is needed for full function

5. **Regarding the elbow, which one of the following statements is FALSE?**
   a. The medial collateral ligament (MCL) is made up of two bands connected by a triangular band
   b. The radial head is a secondary stabiliser to valgus stress
   c. The posterior oblique band of the MCL is only tight when elbow is flexed
   d. The carrying angle increases with flexion of the elbow
   e. The carrying angle should be measured in full extension

6. **Which one of the following best describes the movement at the wrist joint?**
   a. Movement is in two degrees of freedom
   b. The movements of extension and radial deviation are coupled as are flexion and ulnar deviation
   c. Most of "wrist flexion" occurs at the radiocarpal joint
   d. Most "wrist extension" takes place at the midcarpal joint
   e. During radial and ulnar deviation of the wrist the distal carpal row moves in the direction of hand movement

7. **Which of the following best describes the stability and movement of the wrist joint?**
   a. The stability of the wrist joint is mainly bony
   b. Palmar ligaments contribute more to stability than dorsal ligaments
   c. Palmar ligaments resist hyperflexion
   d. During radial deviation the scaphoid extends
   e. During ulnar deviation the lunate flexes

8. **Which of the following best describes the loading of the native human acetabulum?**
   a. Peak compressive forces occur at the supero-lateral labrum
   b. Tensile forces are seen in the posterior wall and compressive forces on the antero-medial side of the hip during heel strike
   c. Compressive forces act predominantly at the posterior and superior acetabulum with tensile stresses acting predominantly on the medial wall
   d. Compressive forces act predominantly at the medial and superior 'weight bearing' dome of the acetabulum
   e. All of the acetabulum is under compressive loads during the stance phase of gait

9. **Which of the following is INCORRECT about the alignment of the knee joint?**
   a. The tibial plateau has a posterior slope of approximately 7°
   b. The normal tibial joint angle is 3° valgus to the mechanical axis of the tibia
   c. The lateral femoral condyle is smaller than the medial
   d. The anatomical tibiofemoral angle is approximately 6° valgus
   e. In a varus knee the weight bearing line falls medial to the centre of the knee joint

10. **Which of the following is INCORRECT about the functional anatomy of the knee joint?**
    a. The surface of the medial tibial plateau is concave
    b. The surface of the lateral tibial plateau is convex
    c. The ACL has anterolateral and posteromedial bands
    d. The PCL has anterolateral and posteromedial bands
    e. The medial meniscus is more tethered than the lateral meniscus

11. **Which of the following best describes the movement at the knee joint?**
    a. The movement of the knee joint occurs in three degrees of freedom
    b. Rotation of the knee joint is unaffected by the degree of knee flexion
    c. Anteroposterior translation of the knee joint is not determined by the degree of knee flexion
    d. The PCL is best assessed at 30° of flexion
    e. The ACL is best assessed at 30° of flexion

12. **Which of the following best describes the movement at the knee joint?**
    a. With knee flexion the medial femoral condyle moves more than the lateral
    b. Knee flexion is performed only by rolling motion
    c. Knee flexion is accompanied by external rotation of the tibia
    d. The medial femoral condyle translates maximally after 120° of knee flexion
    e. There is less than 10° of tibiofemoral rotation in the normal knee during flexion

13. **Which one of the following is the best description of knee ligamentous stability?**
    a. The ACL has the greatest tensile strength of all of the knee ligaments
    b. The deep MCL is the primary restraint to valgus stress
    c. The medial meniscus contributes little to knee stability
    d. The cruciate ligaments are primary stabilisers to tibial rotation
    e. The cruciate ligaments are secondary restraints to varus stress

14. **Which one of the following best describes features of the ACL?**
    a. The ACL receives its innervation from the peroneal nerve
    b. The posterolateral bundle controls anteroposterior translation more than the anteromedial bundle
    c. ACL injuries are more common in male athletes
    d. The posterolateral bundle is tight in knee flexion
    e. In flexion the femoral insertion point of the posterolateral bundle moves anteriorly

15. **Which of the following is INCORRECT about spinal movements?**
    a. Range of flexion increases going from thoracic to lumbar regions
    b. Range of rotation decreases going from thoracic to lumbar regions
    c. Motion within the spine can be described as being 'coupled'
    d. Each intervertebral joint has six degrees of freedom
    e. A motion segment is a vertebra and its named intervertebral disc

16. **Which one of the following is INCORRECT about spinal movements?**
    a. The facet joints and the intervertebral disc determine the range of movement of the spine
    b. Going from cervical to lumbar the angle of the facet joints in the transverse plane increases
    c. Going from cervical to lumbar the angle of the facet joints in the frontal plane increases
    d. Loading of the facet joints is greatest with flexion of the spine
    e. The motion segment exhibits viscoelastic behaviour

17. **In which position is the lumbar (L3) intradiscal pressure the greatest?**
    a. Standing
    b. Bending forwards while standing
    c. Lying
    d. Sitting
    e. Sitting flexed forwards

18. **Which of the following best describes the change in loading of the human acetabulum after conventional metal head on cemented polyethylene cup?**
    a. Increased stresses on the roof and medial wall
    b. Increased stresses on the roof and decreased stresses on the medial wall
    c. Decreased stresses on the roof and increased stresses on the medial wall
    d. Decreased stresses on the roof and medial wall
    e. No change in stress distribution or quantity

19. **Which of the following best describes the change in loading of the human acetabulum with the use of a cemented metal backed polyethylene component compared to a cemented polyethylene cup?**

   a. Increased stresses on the roof and medial wall
   b. Increased stresses on the roof and decreased stresses on the medial wall
   c. Decreased stresses on the roof and increased stresses on the medial wall
   d. Decreased stresses on the roof and medial wall
   e. No change in stress distribution or quantity

20. **A medial opening wedge high tibial osteotomy performed for medial compartmental knee osteoarthritis aims to correct which of the following measurements of axis:**

   a. The weightbearing axis to a point on the lateral tibial plateau that is a maximum of 62.5% of the width of the tibial plateau
   b. The weightbearing axis to a point on the medial tibial plateau that is a maximum of 62.5% of the width of the tibial plateau
   c. The anatomical axis to a point on the lateral tibial plateau that is a maximum of 62.5% of the width of the tibial plateau
   d. The femorotibial mechanical axis to a point on the lateral tibial plateau that is a maximum of 62.5% of the width of the tibial plateau
   e. The femorotibial mechanical axis to a point on the medial tibial plateau that is a maximum of 62.5% of the width of the tibial plateau

21. **Which of the following is NOT a prerequisite for thick film lubrication?**

   a. Low surface roughness
   b. Radial clearance of $>50\ \mu m$
   c. High lambda ratio
   d. High surface wettability
   e. Metal-on-metal articulation

22. **Which of the following statements best describes the relationship between the joint reaction force and the biomechanical environment of the replaced hip?**

    a. Medialisation of the abductors, increased abductor tension, decreased offset and increased leg length all increase joint reaction force
    b. Medialisation of the abductors, increased abductor tension, increased offset and increased leg length all decrease joint reaction force
    c. Lateralisation of the abductors, increased abductor tension (but not decreased offset) and increased leg length all increase joint reaction force
    d. Lateralisation of the abductors, increased abductor tension (but not increased offset) and increased leg length all decrease joint reaction force
    e. Joint reaction force is not determined by hip position following hip arthroplasty

23. **Which one of the following is NOT required to produce the 'hoop stresses' and controlled collapse associated with taper slip prostheses?**

    a. A smooth polished tapered stem
    b. A complete cement mantle
    c. An intact calcar
    d. Viscous cement which is subject to viscoelastic properties
    e. A functioning cement restrictor

24. **Which of the following best describes the effect of increasing the size of a polyethylene cemented cup?**

   a. Increased polyethylene thickness results in increased conformity of the cup increasing the risk of deformity related stress shielding. Increased radius increases angular torque at the cement bone interface and increases the risk of cement interface failure

   b. Increased polyethylene thickness results in decreased conformity of the cup increasing the risk of stress shielding. Increased radius increases angular torque at the cement bone interface and increases the risk of cement interface failure

   c. Increased polyethylene thickness results in increased conformity of the cup increasing the risk of deformity related stress shielding. Increased radius decreases the chances of creep occurring further increasing the rate of loosening

   d. Increased polyethylene thickness results in decreased conformity of the cup increasing the risk of stress shielding. Increased radius decreases the chances of creep occurring further increasing the rate of loosening

   e. The width of the polyethylene has no biomechanical consequences but increasing the width of the polyethylene resists penetrative wear for longer

25. **A patient presents with a fracture of a Charnley stem, proximal to the tip. The implant is well fixed distally. This represents which type of Gruen's failure?**

   a. Type Ia
   b. Type Ib
   c. Type II
   d. Type III
   e. Type IV

26. A patient presents to clinic several years after having undergone a metal-on-polyethylene total hip replacement. He has experienced acute pain and sudden shortening of the leg, and now walks with a 'grating' noise. Radiographs demonstrate that the head is articulating with the outer metal shell of his acetabular component. Which of the following best describes this mode of failure?

    a. Macroscopic polyethylene failure with mode 1 wear
    b. Macroscopic polyethylene failure with mode 2 wear
    c. Macroscopic polyethylene failure with mode 3 wear
    d. Macroscopic polyethylene failure with mode 4 wear
    e. Microscopic polyethylene failure with mode 1 wear
    f. Microscopic polyethylene failure with mode 2 wear
    g. Microscopic polyethylene failure with mode 3 wear
    h. Microscopic polyethylene failure with mode 4 wear

27. Which of the following steps will NOT increase primary arc range hip stability?

    a. Matching of the primary arc range of the replaced and native hip
    b. Increasing the head-neck ratio
    c. Provision of a sub-hemispherical cup
    d. Increasing head size and jump distance
    e. Chamfering the edges of the inner surface of the acetabular component

28. Uncemented metal backed modular acetabular components have been associated with a number of positive and negative effects. When paired to a polyethylene liner which of the following has NOT been associated with uncemented as opposed to cemented monobloc components?

    a. Modulus mismatch between the shell and liner raising the potential for mode 4 wear
    b. Improved survivorships in many joint registries in the younger populations
    c. Lower wear rates when mated to a cross linked polyethylene acetabular component
    d. A lower rate of stress shielding and subsequent better longer lasting 'biological' fixation
    e. May achieve primary fixation with rim expansion

29. With regards to total knee replacements which one of the following statements concerning constraint and wear is INCORRECT?

a. Rotating platform knees are highly constrained, but decrease wear by decoupling forces

b. Medial pivot knees have uniformly higher constraint and consequently lower wear rates than traditional knee replacements

c. Posterior stabilised knees are more highly constrained than PCL retaining knees, but suffer from higher wear rates due to the 'post-cam' articulation

d. Poorly constrained knees may offer higher ranges of motion but suffer from paradoxical sliding and subsequent higher macroscopic wear rates

e. Additional constraint results in higher transmission of torque forces to bone-cement interfaces, but potentially lower abraded wear debris at the articulating surfaces due to lower contact pressures and more congruent articulations

30. With regards to conformity and contact stresses in the knee, which one of the following statements is TRUE?

a. Flat femoral condyle designs mated to flat tibial articulations result in lower contact stresses, and more physiological motion

b. Flat femoral condyle designs mated to flat tibial articulations result in lower contact stresses, and deeper flexion can be achieved due to greater roll back

c. Increasing depth in the same size of polyethylene increases subsurface contact stress concentrations which may result in catastrophic failure of the polyethylene in the presence of normal contact stresses

d. Highly conforming curved surfaces provide the lowest contact stresses and subsequently the lowest chance of subsurface stress concentration, delamination and catastrophic failure

e. Highly conforming curved surfaces provide the highest contact stresses and subsequently the lowest chance of subsurface stress concentration, delamination and catastrophic failure

31. **Which one of the following statements, concerning the design of mobile bearing knee prostheses, most accurately describes the tribological argument for their use?**

    a. The decoupling of shear forces may prevent macroscopic failure of the polyethylene
    b. The rotating platform confers beneficial properties by allowing for 'self-alignment' of tibial rotation and optimisation of patella tracking
    c. The higher conformity of the femoral articulation does not transmit shear forces to the tibia due to the second rotating articulation
    d. Stress applied to polyethylene (PE) in a uniplanar direction results in alignment of the polyethylene chains, loss of PE to adhesive wear and a form of work hardening increasing the resistance to abrasive wear
    e. Mobile bearing knee replacements are similar in design to rotating hinge prostheses

32. **Regarding total knee replacement, what is the minimum thickness of polyethylene spacer that can be implanted whilst avoiding delamination due to the modulus mismatch between the polyethylene and the tibial base plate?**

    a. 4 mm
    b. 6 mm
    c. 8 mm
    d. 10 mm
    e. 12 mm

33. **Which is an appropriate order of soft tissue releases to correct for a fixed varus deformity?**

    a. Superficial MCL, PCL, posteromedial corner, deep MCL
    b. Deep MCL, posteromedial corner, superficial MCL, PCL
    c. Deep MCL, popliteus, posteromedial corner, superficial MCL, PCL
    d. PCL, superficial MCL, popliteus, posteromedial corner, deep MCL, PCL
    e. PCL, deep MCL, popliteus, posteromedial corner, superficial MCL

34. A patient undergoing total knee replacement has 15° of fixed valgus preoperatively. After trial implantation of a cruciate retaining prosthesis, a non-correctable valgus deformity of 12° is identified, worst in extension. The next correct step is:

a. Serial soft tissue releases of : Lateral capsule, ITB, popliteus, LCL, gastrocnemius

b. Serial soft tissue releases of : Lateral capsule, popliteus, ITB, LCL, gastrocnemius

c. Serial soft tissue releases of : Lateral capsule, ITB, popliteus, gastrocnemius, LCL

d. Removal of prosthesis, recutting of the tibia to correct valgus and use of a PCL substituting prosthesis

e. Removal of prosthesis, recutting of the femur to correct valgus and use of a PCL substituting prosthesis

35. Assuming no significant bone loss, when determining the correct rotational orientation for the femoral component in total knee replacement, which one of the following is CORRECT?

a. Whiteside's line is at 90° to the posterior condylar axis, which is itself in 3° of internal rotation relative to the transepicondylar axis

b. Whiteside's line is at 90° to the posterior condylar axis, which is itself in 3° of external rotation relative to the transepicondylar axis

c. Whiteside's line is at 90° to the transepicondylar axis, which is itself in 3° of internal rotation relative to the posterior condylar axis

d. Whiteside's line is at 90° to the transepicondylar axis, which is itself in 3° of external rotation relative to the posterior condylar axis

e. Whiteside's line is at 90° to the anteroposterior axis, and is in 3° of external rotation relative to the posterior condylar axis

36. **What is the definition of the Q angle, and what is its signifi-cance to patellar tracking during knee arthroplasty?**
    a. The angle formed between the direction of pull of the vastus medialis and the patellar tendon. It defines the resultant force on the patella and maximising the Q angle will optimise tracking
    b. The angle formed between the directions of pull of the quadriceps and the patellar tendon. It defines the resultant force on the patella and minimising the Q angle will optimise tracking
    c. The angle formed between the ASIS and the patellar tendon. It defines the resultant force on the patella and maximising the Q angle will optimise tracking
    d. The angle formed between the ISIS and the patellar tendon. It defines the resultant force on the patella and minimising the Q angle will optimise tracking
    e. The angle formed between the ISIS and the patellar tendon. It defines the resultantforce on the patella and maximising the Q angle will optimise tracking

37. **Which of the following correctly describes backside (mode 4) wear in total knee replacement?**
    a. Wear occurring when patients are in deep flexion or "on their backsides". This is particularly a problem in communities where eating sitting on haunches is commonplace
    b. Wear of the articulating femoral component against the "back side" of the tibial tray, when macroscopic failure has occurred
    c. Wear of the "back side" of the patella against the trochlear groove results in anterior knee pain
    d. Posterior condylar wear in deep flexion known as the "lift off – slam down" sequence is also known as "back side" wear
    e. Wear of the non-articulating "backside" of the tibial tray insert. This has been implicated in macroscopic failure of the polyethylene

38. Which one of the following design features will minimise the probability of prosthesis loosening following total knee replacement?

a. A flexible implant with a low thickness to length ratio

b. A titanium tibial baseplate to reduce modulus mismatch at the prosthesis-cement-bone junction on the tibial side alone

c. A square condylar design with low contact area designed to maximise "roll-back"

d. Thin polyethylene to reduce joint reaction forces and the risk of 'sub surface oxidation' and white line formation

e. Peripheral tibial pegs to control rotational torque

39. The biomechanical principle of a "reversed shoulder" arthroplasty refers to:

a. A method of reversing a sided humeral component and using it in a contralateral shoulder to address significant glenoid anteversion

b. Use of a resurfacing arthroplasty with an extended articulating surface to allow for articulation against the acromion in cuff deficient shoulders

c. The practice of cuff interposition arthroplasty at the time of shoulder replacement, thus 'inverting' the polarity of the shoulder

d. An inverse polarity shoulder replacement, designed to provide a glenoid fixed fulcrum for activation of deficient cuff or deltoid muscles with a biomechanical advantage over additional designs

e. An inverse polarity shoulder replacement, designed to provide a humeral fixed fulcrum for activation of deficient cuff or deltoid muscles with a biomechanical advantage over traditional designs

40. Which of the following descriptions best describes the 'sloppy hinge' concept in elbow arthroplasty?

    a. An un-constrained prosthesis that may substitute for collateral incompetence and surgical mal-alignment and reduce transmitted torque forces to either side of the prosthesis. Soft tissue balancing is required

    b. A semi-constrained prosthesis that may substitute for collateral incompetence and surgical mal-alignment and reduce transmitted torque forces to either side of the prosthesis. Soft tissue balancing is required

    c. A constrained prosthesis that may substitute for collateral incompetence and surgical mal-alignment and reduce transmitted torque forces to either side of the prosthesis. The prosthesis is linked but still requires soft tissue balancing

    d. An un-constrained prosthesis that may substitute for collateral incompetence and surgical mal-alignment and reduce transmitted torque forces to either side of the prosthesis. The prosthesis is linked and does not require soft tissue balancing

    e. A semi-constrained prosthesis that may substitute for collateral incompetence and surgical mal-alignment and reduce transmitted torque forces to either side of the prosthesis. The prosthesis is linked and does not require soft tissue balancing

Extended Matching Questions

SCENARIO I OPTIONS

A Radial-collateral ligament
B Lateral ulnar collateral ligament
C Annular ligament
D Anterior oblique bundle of medial collateral ligament
E Posterior oblique bundle of medial collateral ligament
F Transverse medial collateral ligament
G Accessory lateral collateral ligament

This question concerns ligamentous injuries to the elbow. For each of the following injury mechanisms, select from the options above, the ligament most likely to be injured. Each option may be used once, more than once, or not at all.

1. A 70-year-old patient falls to his outstretched hand. He does not sustain a fracture but the ambulance crew report that they 'straightened' his dislocated elbow. In theatre an MUA is performed, during which the patient is demonstrated to have instability in extension and valgus stress.

2. A young man presents with symptoms of instability following an injury whilst ice skating a few months previously. He complains of pain and an unstable feeling in his elbow, particularly when doing push ups.

3. A patient presents three months following a fracture dislocation of his elbow treated operatively, complaining of instability. The patient had a radial head excision and on review of their operative films stress views taken in extension appear unremarkable.

SCENARIO II OPTIONS

A Use of posterior lip
augmentation device (PLAD)
B Trochanteric advancement
C Captured cup

D Increased femoral offset
E Increased head size
F Correction of femoral version
G Correction of cup version

The following clinical case vignettes all concern total hip replacement (THR) instability. For each, select from the options above the most appropriate surgical option for improving hip stability. Each option may be used once, more than once, or not at all.

4. A 70-year-old lady has previously had a stable THR. However, a major CVA leaves her with flaccid paraparesis, following which she develops multi-directional instability of her hip.

5. During THR, stability is assessed intraoperatively with a trial head but with the remainder of both components already in situ. The 'shuck test' is strongly positive, and multidirectional instability is demonstrated, including instability in abduction.

6. A patient complains of post-operative instability following THR through a direct lateral approach. He has had several episodes of dislocation, all when rising from the toilet. Radiographs show a mildly retroverted acetabular component and 25° of anteversion of the femoral stem.

SCENARIO III OPTIONS

A Increase the distal femoral cut

B Downsize the femoral component

C Increase the tibial cut

D Increase the size of the polyethylene

E Increase the size of the femoral component

F Remove posterior osteophytes

G Decrease the size of the tibial polyethylene

This question concerns soft tissue balancing during total knee replacement. For each of the following scenarios, select from the options above, the most appropriate next operative step. Each option may be used once, more than once or not all.

7. Following initial cuts and trialling with a size 8mm tibial insert, the knee is found to be tight in extension, with 5° of fixed flexion, but is balanced otherwise.

8. Following preparation of the bone surfaces the patient is found to be tight in flexion, but not in extension.

9. Following initial bone cuts and trialling with a 12mm tibial spacer the patient is found to be tight in flexion and extension.

SCENARIO IV OPTIONS

A Iliopsoas tendonitis

B Ceramic-ceramic squeak

C Aseptic lymphocyte
   dominated vasculitis
   associated lesion (ALVAL)

D Abrasive wear

E Phase transformation

F Adhesive wear

G Osteolysis

This question concerns possible complications that may occur following total hip replacement. For each of the following scenarios, select the most likely underlying diagnosis from the options above. Each option may be used once, more than once, or not at all.

10. A patient with a ceramic on ceramic articulation sustains a minor stumble off a kerb. The ceramic articulation fractures with a loud noise.

11. During acetabular component revision for aseptic loosening, a 58 mm uncemented cup with a polyethylene liner is inserted. The patient subsequently complains of persistent groin pain. Inflammatory markers are normal; however, on examination the patient experiences pain on resisted flexion and external rotation.

12. A 70-year-old female patient re-presents with pain 2 years following her hip resurfacing procedure. Radiographs do not show any loosening or fracture although she has a small hemi-pelvis and consequently a cup abduction angle of 65°.

SCENARIO V OPTIONS

A	body weight	**E**	5 times body weight
B	2.5 times body weight	**F**	6 times body weight
C	3 times body weight	**G**	7 times body weight
D	4 times body weight	**H**	8 times body weight

Which of the above responses gives the most appropriate value for the following? Each option may be used once, more than once, or not at all.

13. The joint reaction force though the patellofemoral joint when ascending stairs.

14. The joint reaction force though the patellofemoral joint when squatting.

15. The joint reaction force though the tibiofemoral joint when walking.

16. The joint reaction force though the hip joint when walking.

17 The joint reaction force though the tibiotalar joint when walking on flat ground.

Answers: Chapter 14

MCQ 40
EMQ 17

Multiple Choice Answers

1.   A   The position described is O'Brien's test. It is designed to displace the biceps tendon medially and inferiorly and puts strain on the superior labrum and biceps origin. It is a test used clinically to diagnose a SLAP tear.

2.   C   The humeral articular surface is angled 45° superiorly and retroverted 30° with respect to the condylar axis of the humerus. The glenoid is tilted superiorly by 5° and retroverted 7° with respect to the plane of the scapula. The scapula plane is approximately 30° to 50° anterior to the coronal plane of the body. As the armis abducted, two thirds of the motion occurs at the glenohumeral joint and one third occurs at the scapulothoracic joint.

3.   C   The movement of the glenohumeral joint is rotational with approximately 3 mm of superior translation. Anterior ligaments (notably the anterior band of the inferior glenohumeral ligament) are tight in external rotation. Deficiency of the anterosuperior labrum in association with a cord-like MGHL is a normal anatomical variant – the so called Buford complex. Abduction is initiated by supraspinatus before deltoid takes over and becomes more effective with abduction.

4. C The potential number of degrees of freedom in any joint is six. These are AP translation, medio-lateral translation and proximo-distal translation. There is also flexion-extension, internal-external rotation and abduction-adduction.

The elbow theoretically has two degrees of freedom: flexion-extension and pronation-supination. Flexion-extension occurs around an axis through the centre of the trochlea. (In reality other degrees of freedom may also exist, e.g. varus/valgus.)

The MCL is composed of the anterior oblique, posterior oblique and interconnecting transverse ligament. The anterior oblique fibres are tight through the whole range of movement and the posterior oblique fibres are only taut in flexion. It is the primary stabiliser to valgus and rotational stress.

The lateral collateral ligament (LCL) and anconeus provide between 10–15% of the restraint for varus stress. The vast majority is contributed by joint congruity.

The range of movement needed for activities of daily living are between 30° and 130° extension to flexion and 50° of pronation and supination.

5. D The carrying angle is measured in full extension and full supination. It is formed between the intersection of the long axis of the humerus and the long axis of the forearm (although definitions do vary, resulting in different measurements). The angle is approximately 7° in men and 13° in women. The angle decreases with elbow flexion. The radial head is a secondary stabiliser to valgus stress and acts as an important stabiliser when the MCL is incompetent.

6. E There are three degrees of wrist joint movement. The carpus demonstrates coupled motion with the radiocarpal joint. During radial deviation of the radiocarpal joint the proximal row of carpal bones flexes, and during ulnar deviation of the radiocarpal joint they extend. At the radiocarpal joint there is almost twice as much ulnar deviation (40°) compared with radial deviation (20°). During this motion the distal carpal row follows the direction of the fingers whereas the proximal carpal row moves in the opposite direction.

60% of 'wrist flexion' occurs at the midcarpal joint with the rest occurring at the radiocarpal joint. The reverse is true for 'wrist extension', with approximately 67% occurring at radiocarpal joint and the rest occurring at the midcarpal joint.

7. B The stability of the wrist joint is primarily ligamentous. There are palmar and dorsal ligaments and intrinsic and extrinsic ligaments. The palmar ligaments are the strongest and function to resist wrist hyperextension.

With radial deviation of the wrist joint the scaphoid contacts the radial styloid which forces it to flex. This motion is transmitted via the scapholunate ligament to the proximal carpal row, therefore radial deviation of the wrist flexes scaphoid and lunate; during ulnar deviation both bones extend.

8. C In the native hip transmission of compressive forces occurs to the superior and posterior acetabular wall and tensile stresses to the medial wall. After conventional total hip replacement compressive forces on the roof are increased as well as both tensile and compressive stresses in the medial wall.

9. B The tibial plateau has a posterior slope of approximately 7° to 9°. The tibial plateau is in 3° of varus relative to the tibial axis. The lateral femoral condyle is smaller in all dimensions than the medial femoral condyle. The distal femoral condylar axis is 9° valgus with respect to the femoral anatomical axis. Therefore the normal anatomical tibiofemoral angle (the angle between the tibial and femoral anatomical axis) is 6° of valgus.

A valgus deformity is a tibiofemoral angle greater than 6°; a varus angle is a tibiofemoral angle less than 6°.

The weight bearing axis is a line drawn from the centre of the femoral head to the centre of the ankle joint, which in a neutrally aligned limb will fall through the centre of the knee. In a varus knee the weightbearing axis falls to the medial side of the centre of the knee joint, and vice versa with a valgus knee.

10. C The surfaces of the tibial plateaus are asymmetric. The medial plateau is concave whereas the lateral is convex. The menisci serve to create congruency with the femoral condyles. ACL bands are anteromedial and posterolateral (mnemonic – AMPL), PCL bands are anterolateral and posteromedial. The lateral meniscus moves more during knee motion than the medial, which by comparison is relatively tethered.

11. **E** There are theoretically six degrees of freedom in the tibiofemoral joint: flexion-extension rotation around the anatomical axis of the tibia, varus/valgus movement, anteroposterior translation, longitudinal distraction and medial/lateral translation. Rotation of the tibia is affected by the degree of knee extension, with much greater rotation possible in knee flexion (maximum at 90°) and essentially abolished in knee extension. The Lachman test assesses the AP translation of the knee at 30°, the position of maximal AP translation and limited by the ACL. The PCL is assessed at 90° of knee flexion when it should be taut.

12. **D** The flexion of the knee is a complicated combination of rolling and sliding motions of the two femoral condyles. With knee flexion from full extension to 120° the lateral femoral condyle 'rolls back' posteriorly whereas the medial femoral condyle hardly moves. Therefore this movement is associated with 20° of femoral external rotation.

From 120° to full flexion both femoral condyles move a similar amount posteriorly.

Johal P et al. Tibio-femoral movement in the living knee. A study of weight bearing and non-weight bearing knee kinematics using 'interventional' MRI.J Biomech.2005 Feb;38(2):269–76

13. **E** The MCL is the strongest ligament, being almost twice as strong as the other ligaments. The other ligaments are of a similar strength. The cruciates are secondary restraints to tibial rotation and varus/valgus angulation. The superficial MCL is the primary stabiliser to valgus stress and internal rotation. The posterolateral corner, including LCL, is the primary restraint to external rotation.

S.L.-Y. Woo et al. Biomechanics of knee ligaments: injury, healing, and repair. Journal of Biomechanics 39 (2006) 1–20

14. **E**   The ACL is composed of two bundles, a smaller anteromedial bundle and a larger posterolateral bundle, and receives its innervation from the tibial nerve. The AM bundle is tight in flexion and the PL tight in extension (and internal rotation). As the AM bundle tightens the PL bundle loosens.

The AM bundle contributes more to AP translation (Lachman test) than the PL bundle. The PL bundle controls rotation (pivot shift) more than the AM bundle. With knee flexion the PL bundle insertion on the femur is seen to move anteriorly.

Christel P. The contribution of each anterior cruciate ligament bundle to the Lachman test: a cadaver investigation J Bone Joint Surg Br Jan 2012 vol. 94–B no. 1 68–74

15. **E**   Each intervertebral joint possesses a possible six degrees of freedom, with three degrees in translation and three in rotation. These motions are coupled to allow simultaneous translation and rotation. With progression from thoracic to lumbar regions there is an increase in the range of flexion and extension and a decrease in the degree of rotation. A motion segment is defined as two adjacent vertebrae, the shared intervertebral disc and the associated ligaments.

16. **D**   The posterior elements of the spine determine the degree of movement. The loads applied to the facet joints are greatest with extension of the spine.

The orientation of the facet joints changes from cranial to caudal in the transverse and frontal planes. C1 and C2 are exceptional and have facets parallel to the transverse plane. The facets of the rest of the cervical vertebrae are parallel in the frontal plane and 45° in the transverse plane.

The facets of the thoracic vertebrae are orientated 20° in the frontal plane and 60° in the transverse plane.

The facets of the lumbar vertebrae are 45° in the frontal plane and 90° in the transverse plane.

The facets of lumbosacral junction are obliquely orientated to allow some rotation.

As the intervertebral disc is part of the motion segment, the motion segment will exhibit viscoelastic behaviour.

17. **E** The intra discal pressures in L3 are greatest when sitting forwards

The relative intradiscal pressures are as follows (these values are ratios to standing intradiscal pressure):

Lying – 0.75

Standing – 1

Bending forwards while standing – 1.5

Bending forwards while standing with weights in the hands – 2.2

Sitting – 1.4

Sitting flexed forwards – 1.85

Sitting flexed forwards with weights in the hands – 2.75

Other authors have found similar findings for lying, standing but some have shown the highest values to be when bending forwards with a weight in the hands

A.L. Nachemson, Spine 1976, 1 pp. 59–71

Wilke H. New in vivo measurements of pressures in the intervertebral disc in daily life. Spine (Phila Pa 1976)1999 Apr 15;24(8):755–62

18. **A** In the native hip there is transmission of compressive stresses to the superior and posterior acetabular wall and tensile stresses to the medial wall. After conventional total hip replacement there are tension-compression stresses in the medial wall of the acetabulum and large tensile stresses in the roof and inferior margin of the cup.

Vasu R J. Stress distributions in the acetabular region—I. Before and after total joint replacement. Biomech. 1982;15(3):155–64

19. **D** The addition of a 2 mm cobalt chrome metal back to the polyethylene cup leads to a decrease in the stresses in cement and bone compared with a polyethylene cup with no metal back. However, this of course does not translate into better clinical results

Carter D et al. Stress distributions in the acetabular region-II. Effects of cement thickness and metal backing of the total hip acetabular component. J.Biomech. 1982;15(3):165–70.

20.   A   A medial opening wedge HTO aims to alter the weightbearing axis away from the diseased medial compartment and into the lateral compartment. The maximum movement should be to 62.5% of the width of the tibial plateau towards the lateral side; this is known as Fujisawa's point.

If there is lateral compartmental disease then the degree of correction can be titrated more towards to the midline.

Birmingham et al. Medial Opening Wedge High Tibial Osteotomy: A Prospective Cohort Study of Gait, Radiographic, and Patient-Reported Outcomes. Arthritis & Rheumatism (Arthritis Care & Research) Vol. 61, No. 5, May 15, 2009, pp 648–657

21.   E   To achieve thick film (fluid film) lubrication, the pre-requisite is a fluid film thickness greater than the separation between the two surfaces. This requires a high radial clearance and lambda ratio, low surface roughness and high wettability. (The lambda ratio refers to the ratio of the fluid film thickness to the surface roughness; for thick film lubrication this should be above 3.) Although metal-on-metal articulations are often implicated in thick film lubrication it can also occur with ceramic-on-ceramic bearings.

22.   A   The abductors provide the major force on the hip following a total joint arthroplasty. Decreasing the lever arm or offset or increasing abductor tension will increase the work the muscles have to do, and consequently their contribution to the joint reaction force. Leg lengthening occurs within the hip itself and is akin to an abductor lengthening.

23.   C   An intact calcar is not required for taperslip hip replacements which may therefore be used with calcar deficiency or fracture. A taperslip prosthesis requires a smooth polished stem implanted inside an intact cortex using viscous cement with properties of creep. The Swedish joint registry demonstrates higher failure rates with cemented stems when a cement restrictor (or bone block is not used). RSA studies have demonstrated that a cement restrictor is critical to the classic 'controlled migration' associated with a taper slip stem.

24. B Increasing the radius of a cemented cup increases the effective lever arm and consequently the angular torque from friction at the head cup interface. Increased thickness results in a stiffer cup with greater potential for stress shielding. Increased thickness of the cup does not affect the ability of polyethylene to creep as this is a material property.

25. E The question describes cantilever bending which is type IV. Gruen's defined types of failure are:

Type	Failure Mode
Ia	Pistoning (stem-cement interface)
Ib	Pistoning (cement-bone interface)
II	Midstem pivot
III	Calcar pivot
IV	Cantilever failure

26. B This scenario describes macroscopic failure of the polyethylene liner as the polyethylene has lost its structural integrity. It is type 2 wear (see below).

Mode of wear	Description
1	Generation of wear debris between two intended articulating surfaces
2	Generation of wear debris between an intended and unintended articulation
3	Third body wear between two articulating surfaces
4	Wear between two non-articulating surfaces (e.g. trunion)

27. D Increasing head size in joint arthroplasty increases the stability by increasing the jump distance; however, it does not *per se* increase the primary arc range. It is the head:neck ratio that determines the primary arc range, not head size alone.

28. D Solid back metal shell components have been associated with stress shielding and subsequent relative osteopaenia. Although 'biologic' fixation is associated with porous coated prosthesis, the rates of stress shielding are higher than in cemented monobloc components.

29. B The medial pivot knee is highly constrained and has conforming polyethylene in the medial compartment, but lower conformity and constraint in the lateral compartment designed to mirror more closely the normal biomechanics of a human knee than traditional resurfacing designs.

30. D High conformity reduces contact stresses and therefore the chances of catastrophic failure. Flattening the femoral condyles does reduce the contact stresses, but can result in paradoxical motion, and reduces stability in the coronal and sagittal planes. Increasing the depth of the polyethylene reduces the chances of subsurface delamination from stress concentrations associated with thin poly designs.

31. D Tribological arguments refer specifically to material properties arguments, not biomechanical considerations. Whilst A–C are also valid, they refer to the biomechanics of the joint, not the tribology of the surface. Statement E is incorrect.

32. C 8 mm is the minimum width of polyethylene required to prevent delamination associated with subsurface stress concentration. This is at the deepest point of the dish, so often 10 mm or 12 mm 'sized' spacers will be required to maintain the 8 mm required poly thickness.

33. B Varus releases must start with the most accessible structure first (Deep MCL). The PCL may be released at any point, and may be routinely released with PCL-substituting prostheses. The posteromedial corner should be released before the superficial MCL as this may be associated with iatrogenic instability. The popliteus is not tight in varus knees.

34. A Soft tissue releases are appropriate to correct this deformity. As the patient is tight in extension the ITB (which is tight in extension) should be released before popliteus. Gastrocnemius should be the last release as aggressive release can result in instability and weakness in knee flexion. Whilst some surgeons would advocate the use of a PCL substituting prosthesis for all valgas deformities, a cruciate retaining device is acceptable for smaller deformities.

35. D Whiteside's line is the eponymous name for the antero-posterior axis, and is at a right-angle to the transepicondylar axis. Owing to the larger medial femoral condyle, the transepicondylar axis is slightly externally rotated relative to the posterior condylar axis in the anatomically normal knee; the equal flexion gap in the native knee is maintained by slight varus alignment of the tibial plateau. In total knee replacement the tibia is cut at 90° to the long axis of the tibia; the femoral component must therefore be externally rotated by 3° to maintain the correct flexion gap. This is achieved either by aligning the femoral component rotation with the transepicondylar axis (i.e. at 90° to Whiteside's line), or by externally rotating it by 3° relative to the posterior condylar axis.

36. B The Q angle is the angle formed by the line of pull of the quadriceps (taken as the ASIS radiographically to the middle of the patella) and the patellar tendon (radiographically taken as the tibial tubercle). It determines the resultant force vector on the patella (which usually includes a lateral vector), and thereby its tracking. Minimising the Q angle improves tracking. The ISIS is the origin of one of the heads of rectus and is virtually analogous to the Q-angle, but not the strict definition.

37. E Although all of the scenarios outlined are all problems with total knee replacement, backside (mode 4) wear refers specifically to that occurring between two intentionally non-articulating surfaces; such as that which occurs behind the polyethylene tray insert.

38. B Titanium tibial baseplates are thought to reduce the chances of early loosening associated with cobalt chrome baseplates. All-polyethylene tibial components have not been shown to be associated with any increase in early failure in the older population, but younger patients do not do well with all-polyethylene components in some studies.

39. D An inverse or reverse polarity shoulder simply refers to the fixed fulcrum on the glenoid bone, rather than the humerus. The biomechanical advantages are as stated.

40. E The sloppy hinge does not require ligament balancing, but will substitute for lax or incompetent ligaments. The 'sloppy' refers to a semiconstrained prosthesis which will dissipate some but not all of the torsional forces across the elbow.

Extending Matching Answers

1. D The antero-medial or antero-oblique portion of the medial collateral ligament is the primary stabiliser of the elbow to valgus strain and is most active in extension.

2. B Postero-lateral rotatory instability is associated with LUCL injury and is typically present in deep flexion and external rotation such as when performing press ups.

3. E The radial head an important contributor to stability in flexion with valgus force. The posterior bundle of the medial collateral ligament is tight in flexion. With normal stress views in extension the more commonly injured anterior portion of the MCL must be intact.

4. C The lady has a muscle tone dysfunction and multi-direction instability. Trochanteric advancement is of no benefit if the abductors are not functioning. She therefore requires a captured cup.

5. D The patient has failed the 'shuck test' which tests abductor tone with inline traction. As the implants are already implanted the easiest way to increase abductor tone is to increase femoral neck offset by increasing the head offset. Abductor advancement carries some morbidity and risk of non-union.

6. G Whilst correction of either femoral or acetabular version can be used to correct 'combined version', the femoral component in this case is already significantly anteverted. It is most likely his posterior instability in flexion is due to acetabular component malalignment, and revision of this component is therefore more appropriate.

7. F If the soft tissues are otherwise balanced, then the next step is to remove the posterior osteophytes to correct the fixed flexion deformity. The next step if this fails to address the fix flexion would be to "release" the posterior capsule. The last step is to resect more distal femur; however, this would have the effect of raising the joint line.

8. B When the patient is tight in flexion this means the posterior condyles of the implant are larger than those resected. Hence the patient is tight in flexion. The options are to anteriorly translate the prosthesis (which often results in overstuffing of the patellofemoral joint) or to downsize the femoral component.

9. G Where possible, the orthopaedic surgeon should always attempt to preserve the patient's own bone stock. Although a larger tibial cut will achieve the same as a narrower insert it is more suitable to change the insert and maintain the patient's bone, given that the minimum allowable width of polyethylene is 8mm.

10. E This represents phase transformation which can occur if the ceramic is manufactured with too much moisture. Phase transformed ceramic is brittle and prone to fracture.

11. A Large uncemented cups have been associated with iliopsoas tendonitis, as the large metal shell can irritate the psoas tendon as it passes over the pelvic brim.

12. C The patient has typical symptoms of ALVAL with no radiographic changes but many of the risk factors (open cup, small head size, female sex) and unremarkable radiography. A MARS MRI scan would confirm the diagnosis.

13. B See answer 15 for explanation.

14. H See answer 15 for explanation.

15. B The patella acts to increase the effectiveness of the lever arm of the quadriceps, reportedly by up to 50%. The position of the joint reaction force changes as the knee is flexed. As the patella engages, the inferior pole of the patella contacts the trochlea at approximately 10–20° knee flexion. With increasing knee flexion the position of the joint reaction force moves proximally.

On flat walking the patellofemoral joint reaction force is 0.5 times body weight. This increases to 2.5 times body weight when climbing stairs and 8 times body weight when squatting.

2.5 times body weight passes through the tibiofemoral joint when walking.

Oliver S. Schindler, W. Norman Scott Basic kinematics and biomechanics of the patello-femoral joint Part 1: The native patella Acta Orthop. Belg., 2011, 77, 421–431

D'Lima, The 2011 ABJS Nicolas Andry Award: 'Lab'-in-a-Knee: In Vivo Knee Forces, Kinematics, and Contact Analysis Clin Orthop Relat Res (2011) 469:2953–2970

16. **C** Peak acetabular stress is three times body weight during normal gait. During stair climbing and running this stress increases. This has been both measured directly and derived from free body diagrams.

Bergmann G. Hip contact forces and gait patterns from routine activities. Biomech.2001 Jul;34(7):859–71

17. **E** The ground reaction force through the tibiotalar joint whilst walking on flat ground is reportedly five times body weight. The peak is during the latter part of stance phase.

Stauffer RN, Chao EY, Brewster RC. Force and motion analysis of the normal, diseased,and prosthetic ankle joint.Clin Orthop 1977; 127:189–96

Chapter 15

Perioperative Problems and Theatre Design

MCQ 20
EMQ 4

Multiple Choice Questions

1. The anaesthetic room falls into which of the following categories?

   a. Aseptic
   b. Clean
   c. Clean enclosed
   d. Dirty
   e. Back corridor

2. Which of the following was investigated and found not to reduce post-operative infection rates in the MRC infection trial of joint replacements?

   a. Systemic antibiotics
   b. Topical antibiotics (loaded cement)
   c. Use of vented suits
   d. Use of horizontal laminar flow
   e. Pre-coated cement implants

3. **Which one of the following statements relating to perioperative thromboprophylaxis is TRUE?**
   a. All patients must have extended thromboprophylaxis following total hip replacement
   b. Rivaroxiban is an oral factor Xa inhibitor
   c. Low molecular weight heparin is safe for patient use without monitoring
   d. Patients on warfarin do not need to take other forms of prophylaxis perioperatively
   e. Patients undergoing day case surgery do not need thromboprophylaxis

4. **What is the required light intensity within the operative surgical field?**
   a. 100 lux
   b. 4,000 lux
   c. 8,000 lux
   d. 40,000 lux
   e. 80,000 lux

5. **Which one of the following is responsible for the development of malignant hyperpyrexia?**
   a. Uncontrolled hypothermia due to the effect of suxamethonium inhibition of ion pumps in human mitochondria
   b. Suxamethonium administration in the presence of halothane anaesthetics
   c. Autosomal recessive gene
   d. Autosomal dominant gene
   e. Dantrolene administration in the presence of an x-linked recessive mutation

6. **Without prophylaxis, what is the rate of symptomatic post-operative deep vein thrombosis (DVT) following total hip replacement?**
   a. 0.01%
   b. 0.1%
   c. 1%
   d. 2%
   e. Greater than 10%

7. **Which of the following ventilation systems relies on passive air diffusion?**

    a. Entrainment

    b. Horizonal laminar flow

    c. Vertical laminar flow

    d. Plenium

    e. Houndsfield enclosure

8. **A 'Howorth enclosure' refers to which one of the following?**

    a. A non-rebreathing oxygen mask with controlled oxygen delivery via interchangeable calibrated valves

    b. An inverted trumpet (or exponential airflow) of air generated with a canopy designed to avoid peripheral entrainment

    c. An old-fashioned form of laminar flow with Perspex doors reaching to the theatre floor to avoid turbulent air flow

    d. The closed circuit sterilisation units used in modern theatre suites combining high pressure with moist heat to ensure rapid sterilisation

    e. A form of pudding basin used mostly to make three-tier jelly

9. **Which one of the following most accurately describes the NICE guidance on perioperative thromboprophylaxis?**

    a. Knee arthroscopy – none; total knee replacement – risk score; total hip replacement – risk score

    b. Knee arthroscopy – none; total knee replacement – 2 weeks; total hip replacement – 2 weeks

    c. Knee arthroscopy – risk score; total knee replacement – 4 weeks; total hip replacement – 2 weeks

    d. Knee arthroscopy – risk score; total knee replacement – 2 weeks; total hip replacement – 4 weeks

    e. Knee arthroscopy – risk score; total knee replacement – 4 weeks; total hip replacement – 4 weeks

10. **With regards to post-operative closed suction drains in hip arthroplasty procedures, which one of the following statements is TRUE?**

    a. Retransfusion drains have been shown significantly to reduce the rate of post-operative transfusion following total hip replacement

    b. Post-operative haematoma formation is demonstrably more common without a closed suction drain

    c. Several studies have supported the practice of clamping retransfusion drains for a period of time immediately post-operatively

    d. There is a significant increase in infection rates if drains are left in for greater than 48 hours

    e. There is evidence to support the routine insertion of closed suction drains in hip hemiarthroplasty

11. **Which of the following has been conclusively demonstrated to decrease wound infection post hemiarthroplasty of the hip?**

    a. Subcuticular closure

    b. Four postoperative doses of systemic antibiotics as opposed to three

    c. Use of iodine impregnated 'opsite' adhesive plastic skin drapes

    d. Wound irrigation with antiseptic agents during closure

    e. Use of high pressure pulsed lavage irrigation in the endosteal canal prior to prosthesis implantation

12. **Post-operative pin site infection is a common problem with the use of circular ring fixation. Which one of the following statements is CORRECT?**

    a. Regular swabbing and cleaning of the pin sites with alcohol swabs decrease infection rate

    b. Positioning of half pins in areas with thick soft tissue coverage decreases infection rates

    c. Infection rates are higher in half pins than in fine wire sites

    d. Pin site infection often results in osteomyelitis if not promptly treated

    e. The rate of half pin introduction is accepted to affect the rate of post-operative infection

13. A patient is admitted with an Injury Severity Score of 19. Initial observations and investigations reveal Hb 9.2, pH 7.2, Lactate 3.1, Na$^+$ 132, heart rate 114 and blood pressure 115/53. Which one of the following statements is FALSE?

    a. The patient is currently in stage III shock and should undergo aggressive resuscitation with blood products to maintain end organ perfusion pressure prior to undergoing any surgery

    b. The patient should initially undergo damage control surgery; following the principles of lactate-controlled surgery the patient may return to theatre at any time once the lactate has fallen back to the pre-operative level

    c. Administration of tranexamic acid to the patient will reduce their risk of death

    d. The patient does not have isolated limb injuries and so management should involve a multi-disciplinary approach

    e. There is no place for an early total care approach to reduce secondary physiological stress in patients with such injuries

14. A patient has undergone operative fixation of a segmental humeral fracture, following which she has altered sensation in the hand, active but restricted finger extension, and normal wrist extension. The little finger sits in a slightly abducted position. Grip strength is normal. Which of the following describes the nerve lesion(s)?

    a. Cubital tunnel syndrome

    b. Ulnar nerve intact, radial axonotmesis and median nerves intact

    c. Ulnar nerve intact, radial neuropraxia and median nerves intact

    d. Ulnar nerve neuropraxia, radial and median nerves intact

    e. Ulnar nerve neuropraxia, radial neuropraxia and median nerves intact

15. **What is the % increase in post-operative mortality in patients in whom a myocardial infarction has occurred within the month immediately preceding surgery?**

    a. 50%
    b. 100%
    c. 250%
    d. 400%
    e. 1000%

16. **Which one of the following statements concerning post-operative complications following surgery is FALSE?**

    a. The Thompson's approach is associated with posterior interosseous nerve (PIN) palsy
    b. The Hardinge approach to the hip is not associated with a specific nerve palsy
    c. Rates of dislocation following total hip replacement are higher with the posterior approach
    d. Axillary nerve palsy is associated with the McKenzie approach
    e. The distal Henry approach utilises an inter-nervous plane and may be associated with injury to median or radial nerves

17. **Which one of the following is NOT associated with an above average incidence of hip dislocation of the hip?**

    a. Primary total hip replacement in a patient with a previous history of poliomyelitis
    b. Primary total hip replacement undertaken acutely following intracapsular neck of femur fracture
    c. Primary total hip replacement in a patient with a previous history of cerebrovascular insult
    d. Use of a 'high hip centre' in DDH
    e. Revision large head total hip replacement performed for periprosthetic fracture

18. **Which one of the following is associated with a better than average rate of union if treated surgically?**

    a. A head splitting fracture of the proximal humerus
    b. A four part fracture of the proximal humerus
    c. Yakoub fracture of the proximal humerus
    d. A two part humeral fracture in a patient with myeloma
    e. A varus impacted fracture of the humeral head

19. **Which one of the following is a potential adverse effect of the addition of topical antibiotics to polymethylmethacrylate (PMMA) cement?**

    a. Decreased ductility of the cement
    b. Increased rates of radiolucent lines and early loosening
    c. Thermal necrosis of the surrounding cancellous bone
    d. Failure of polymerisation due to early chain scission and subsequent subsidence of the stem
    e. Higher rates of polyethylene wear due to the increased abrasive nature of the PMMA-particles with antibiotics compared to PMMA without antibiotics

20. **Which one of the following is a contra-indication to the use of a retransfusion drain following joint replacement surgery?**

    a. Macrocytic anaemia
    b. Use of a cemented prosthesis
    c. Second stage revision for infection
    d. Latex allergy
    e. Implantation of a THR for Mirels' grade 7 hip

Extended Matching Questions

SCENARIO I OPTIONS

A Heparin induced thrombocytopaenia. Give protamine

B Acute sickle cell crisis. Give IV saline and dantroline

C Heparin induced thrombocytopaenia. Stop heparin and begin warfarin therapy

D Acute sickle cell crisis. Give IV saline and keep well oxygenated

E Acute bone marrow suppression secondary to trauma. Begin aggressive supportive therapy

F Chronic bone marrow suppression secondary to haemorrhage. Transfuse to physiological status

G Primary iron deficiency anaemia. Treat with oral or IV iron

H Unmasked von Willebrand's disease. Treat expectantly

I Undiagnosed haemophilia B. Treat with factor VIII and transfusion, if required

J Undiagnosed haemophilia B. Treat with factor IX and transfusion, if required

Which of the above diagnoses and treatment options best describes the following case vignettes? Each option may be used once, more than once, or not at all.

1. Following an RTA and surgery for bilateral open femoral fractures you review the patient on ITU and are shown the post-operative blood tests by the nurse:

Hb	7.9
Platelets	204
Fe	130
Ferritin	320
TIBC	341
INR	1.3
APTT	37

'Biphasic waveform noted'

2. You are asked to review an Afro-Carribean who recently had a knee replacement. They have an acutely painful leg and a leaky wound. The surgery was 4 days ago. The patient mentions that they may be a sickle cell carrier and wonders if a new rash on their legs might be a sickle cell crisis. You review their recent blood results:

Hb	12.3
Platelets	120
Fe	121
Ferritin	310
TIBC	370
INR	1.1
APTT	97

3. A previously well 47-year-old male patient has persistent ooze following total hip replacement. Your FY2 has sought haematology advice as they are concerned the patient may have developed HIT due to an expanding haematoma in the patient's leg. They call you with the results of the blood tests the haematologist requested:

Hb	12.3
Platelets	473
INR	1.1
APTT	97
BT	7

4. A previously well 49-year-old female patient persistently attends A&E following day case carpal tunnel decompression with ongoing low grade slow haemorrhagic ooze. On her third attendance she is referred to the orthopaedic on-call team with the following blood results:

Hb	11.2
Platelets	443
INR	1.1
APTT	62
BT	19

Answers: Chapter 15

> **MCQ 20**
> **EMQ 4**

Multiple Choice Answers

1. B Theatre design calls for graded levels of cleanliness, with the theatre and lay-up room being the 'aseptic' area, the rest of the suite 'clean' and the back corridor/sluice the 'dirty' area. Personnel and air flow should take this into account.

2. D The MRC (Lidwell) trial did not examine pre-coated implants. It found laminar flow in general to lower post-operative deep infection rates, but horizontal laminar flow only to be useful in hip arthroplasty, not in other joints. This is probably due to the difficulties with patient positioning.

3. B NICE recommends risk scoring for all patients prior to surgery and thromboprophylaxis for all high risk patients (including day cases) if required. LMWH requires regular platelet checks to ensure the patient has not developed heparin induced thrombocytopenia (HIT). Warfarin must be stopped pre-operatively, and when restarted has a mild pro-coagulant effect due to its greater inhibition of protein C and protein S production within the first 48 hours; LMWH should therefore be co-administered.

4. D 40,000 lux is the recommended light intensity at the surgical site.

5. D Malignant hyperpyrexia (MH) is an autosomal dominant genetic trait resulting in uncontrolled hyperthermia due to an error in mitochondrial function. A variety of mechanisms are implicated but the common pathway is broadly an increase in intracellular calcium within skeletal muscle, with associated myofibril contraction. MH is treated with dantrolene.

6. E Although studies vary, and there is little modern evidence, the majority of data report symptomatic DVT rates of at least 10% in patients without chemo-mechanical prophylaxis. Methods taken to reduce this figure include early mobilisation, hydration, spinal anaesthetic, mechanical prophylaxis and chemical anticoagulation.

7. D   Plenium ventilation relies on filtered air, with higher pressure within the operating theatre than the outer areas. Balanced ventilation ensures one-way airflow. High efficiency particulate arrest filtration (HEPA) ensures that over 99.97% of all particles greater than 0.3μm are removed.

8. B   The Howorth enclosure results in airflow in the shape of an inverted trumpet which helps to avoid entrainment of air from outside the operative field.

9. D   Whilst the NICE guidelines recommend risk scoring every patient, they also recommend at least 2 weeks' thromboprophylaxis following TKR and 4 weeks' after THR. Answer A is incorrect as even daycase arthroscopy must be risk scored.

10. D   Multiple studies have shown an increased rate of post-operative drain contamination when drains are left in for more than 48 hours. There is little evidence for or against the routine use of closed suction drains and consequently all the other statements are false.

11. A   Multiple randomised controlled trials and several meta-analyses have shown a reduction in post-operative wound infection rates with hand sewn subcuticular closure. Endosteal pulsed lavage improves the cement interdigitation with cemented prostheses and the prosthesis-bone interface in uncemented prostheses, but does not decrease post-operative infection rates. Although intuitively the other options seem likely to reduce post-operative infection rates, there is no supporting literature for their use.

12. E   Pin site infections are more common with unstable or loose pins. Meticulous insertion including slow drilling with regular irrigation and slow introduction reduces the thermal necrosis in cortical bone. Excessive thermal necrosis during introduction results in subsequent loss of stability and micro-motion of the half pin resulting in infection. Pin tract infections are more common in areas with thick overlying soft tissue coverage such as the thigh than in subcutaneous bone such as the tibial face.

13. B   The patient has grade III shock and multiple body regions are injured. The reduction of post-operative complications (death, SIRS, ARDS and thromboembolic disease) relies on adequate pre-operative management. Timing of secondary surgery after damage control surgery by lactate should wait until the lactate is less than 2.

Use of an early total care strategy provides the maximal 'second hit' or secondary physiological stress associated with surgery. In order to reduce the second hit a 'damage control approach' is used.

14. D The patient has an intact median nerve as the long flexors are intact. The lack of complete loss of power in wrist extension excludes a radial nerve palsy at the humeral level. A high ulnar nerve lesion results in loss of intrinsic function (extensors) and Wartenberg's escape (abducted little finger). The maintenance of sensation precludes an axonotmesis or neurotmesis.

15. D Rates of mortality are increased by approximately 400% if the patient has had a proven myocardial infarction within the month immediately preceding surgery and are increased 250% within 6 months.

16. B The Hardinge approach is associated with a superior gluteal nerve palsy as the nerve passes through the gluteus medius just proximal to the incision. The Thompson's approach accesses the radius posteriorly and thus may injure the PIN. The posterior approach to the hip is traditionally associated with higher dislocation rates, although this may now be largely historical. McKenzie described an anterosuperior approach to the glenohumeral joint.

17. D Maintenance of a high hip centre is an accepted, although older, approach in DDH surgery. It maintains the natural muscle tension, avoids sciatic nerve traction and maintains bone stock. However, it does not restore leg length or normal hip biomechanics. Revision THR is associated with higher dislocation rates as are all neuro-muscular problems, and complication rates have also been previously shown to be higher following THR for trauma.

18. C The Yakoub fracture of the proximal humerus has an intact medial hinge and varus four part fracture of the proximal humerus which maintains the blood supply. All forms of malignancy potentially reduce rates of union.

19. A Addition of antibiotics can affect the mechanical properties of the cement polymer, which tends to decrease ductility so affecting the ability of the cement to cold flow, thus increasing the likelihood of cement fracture. It has no effect on loosening and decreases the thermal energy released during polymerisation. The barium or zirconium added for radiolucency increase the abrasive nature of cement debris.

20. E Retransfusion drains are contra-indicated in cancer surgery due to the risk of metastatic seeding. They are not contra-indicated in any of the other conditions.

Extending Matching Answers

1. E   The patient is mildly anaemic with somewhat deranged clotting secondary to trauma and subsequent major surgery. The 'biphasic waveform' is pathognomonic for disseminated intravascular coagulopathy (DIC), and supportive therapy should be commenced immediately. The iron/transferrin values are normal. Total iron binding capacity is a measure of nutrition and chronic liver function.

2. C   The patient is mildly thrombcytopaenic, has recently had a knee replacement and will therefore be on LMWH as per NICE guidance. Although a haematology assay (ELIZA) is required to confirm the diagnosis it is likely the patient has heparin induced thrombocytopaenia. The treatment is not to reverse with protamine (due to the increased risk of thrombosis), but rather to anticoagulate with a different agent.

3. J   The patient has an expanding haematoma and a bleeding disorder. The raised APTT and normal bleeding time with normal platelets would suggest a diagnosis of haemophilia. This must be Haemophilia B which may go undiagnosed, and is treated with factor IX if required.

4. H   The patient has had day surgery so will not be on heparin. The increased bleeding time is diagnostic of von Willebrand's disease and can be treated without patient investigation and expectantly in the absence of major haemorrhage.

Index

Note: Only the questions have been indexed and almost all of them come from the main part of the question (in green in the MCQs). These are indexed by chapter and question number followed by the letter M (for MCQ) or E (for EMQ). Chapter topics are indexed by page ranges in **bold**.

lymphocytic vasculitis, aseptic 6.23M

McKenzie approach and nerve injury 15.16M
magnetic resonance imaging (MRI) 2.15M
   dark structures on both T1- and T2-weighted images 2.1M
   proton precession 2.7M
malignant hyperpyrexia 10.8M, 15.5M
malignant tumours (oncology) 10.13–14M
   bone 10.10–12E, 10.21–3M
      secondary (metastases) 10.17M
   soft tissue 10.21M
   synovium 10.19M, 11.1E
Mann–Whitney U-test 12.8–10M
march fracture 9.17M
Marfan syndrome 11.3E
mean 12.21M
   measure of spread about 12.2M
   standard error of 12.21M
median 12.1M, 12.21M
median nerve 1.4M, 1.23M, 1.29M
meiosis 11.11M
Meissner's corpuscles 4.7M
Mendelian inheritance patterns 11.5E
meniscofemoral ligament, posterior (Wrisburg's ligament) 1.16M
meniscus 5.6–10E, 5.20M
   biomechanics 5.15, 14.10M, 14.13M
   damage/tear/injury 5.10E, 5.21–2M
   forces 5.6–8E
   lateral 5.7E
   medial 5.6E, 5.8E, 5.22M
      excision 5.9E
   structure 5.12M
mesenchymal stem cells 10.15E
meta-analysis 12.18M
metacarpal ligament, superficial transverse (natatory ligaments) 1.35M
metacarpophalangeal (MCP) joint extended or flexed, PIP flexion difficulties with 13.4M, 13.5E
metals
   corrosion 8.10M
   total hip replacement
      acetabular 14.28M
      femoral head, advantages of ceramic head over 8.9M
metastases, bone 10.17M
metatarsal break phenomenon 9.17M
metatarsalgia, Morton's (Morton's neuroma) 9.6E
metatarsophalangeal joint extension 9.18M
microscopy see electron microscopy; light microscopy
mode 12.1M, 12.21M
monoclonal antibody therapy, rheumatoid arthritis 6.16M
Morton's neuroma 9.6E
motor neuron injury, upper 4.17M
motor units 4.4M
MRI see magnetic resonance imaging
multiple endocrine neoplasia type I 11.3E

multiple epiphyseal dysplasia 10.27M
multiple injury see injury
muscle (skeletal) **55–75**
muscle fibres, type 1 4.18M
muscle spindles 4.9M
muscle/tendon transfers
   to hand and forearm 4.19M
   from hand for peripheral nerve lesions 13.15M
mutations causing orthopaedic disorders 11.1–5E
Mycobacterium tuberculosis infection 6.4E, 6.14M, 6.27M
myocardial infarction (month preceding surgery), postoperative mortality risk 15.15M
myosin 4.15M, 4.20M

nails, intramedullary 3.5–8E, 3.11M, 3.12–13E
natatory ligaments 1.35M
necrotising fasciitis 6.28–9M
neoplasms see tumours
nerve(s), peripheral **55–75**
   lesions 13.12M
      donor tendons in repair 13.15M
      in humeral fracture 15.14M
   surgical approaches and risk of injury 15.16M
   to cervical vertebra 1.22M
   to pectoralis minor 1.3M
nerve root (radicular) symptoms in legs 1.31M
neural tumours 10.18M
neurofibromatosis 10.18M
neuroma, Morton's 9.6E
neuromuscular transmission 4.11M
neuronal function 4.3M
neurovascular structures see blood supply; nerves
non-parametric data
   average 12.1M
   significant difference analysis 12.13M
notch sensitivity 8.7E
nucleus pulposus 5.14M, 5.17M
null hypothesis 12.16M

Ollier's disease (enchondromatosis) 10.22M, 11.6E
oncology see malignant tumours
operating theatre design **274–88**
orthoses 9.6–10E, 9.10M, 9.15M
Ortolani test 2.1M
ossification
   endochondral 11.19M
   pisiform 11.2M
osteoarthritis 5.11M
   cartilage in 5.4M
   knee 14.20M
   tarsometatarsal 9.9E
osteogenesis imperfecta 5.1E, 10.7M
osteoinductive substances 3.14M
osteolysis 6.25M
   joint replacement and 8.21M
   hip 6.6E
osteomalacia 10.6M
osteomyelitis 6.20M, 10.13E
osteopetrosis 11.9E

osteoporosis
   prevention 10.1E
   WHO definition 2.3M
osteosarcoma incidence 12.3M
osteotomy, opening wedge high tibial
   anterior 7.22M
   medial 14.20M
outcome analysis 12.15M
   randomised controlled trials 12.14M

Pacinian corpuscles 13.13M
paediatrics see children
pagetoid transformation, malignant 10.23M
pain
   low back 1.32M
   radial side of wrist 13.9E
paired Student's T-test 12.6M, 12.8–10M
palmar, see volar
parasympathetic nervous system 4.13M
parathyroid hormone (PTH) 6.8M, 10.5M
passivation of biomaterials 8.12M
Patau syndrome 11.8M
patellar tracking in knee arthroplasty 14.36M
patellofemoral joint reaction forces see reaction forces
pectoralis minor, nerve supply 1.3M
peptidoglycan synthesis inhibitors 6.3M
peripheral nerve see nerve
Perthes' disease 10.6E
pes (talipes) equinovarus 10.29M
PET (positron emission tomography) 2.13M
pharmacology **95–111**
phase transformation 8.18M
phospholipid bilayer 4.7E
physis (growth plate)
   lower limb, in longitudinal growth 11.14M
   Salter–Harris type I fracture 10.14E
   zones 10.9M, 11.13M
      in rickets 10.4M
      in systemic physiological stress 11.3M
pins (for fractures) 3.13M, 6.20M
   postoperative infection at site of 15.12M
pisiform, ossification of 11.2M
pistoning (prosthesis) in swing phase in below knee amputation 9.5M
pivot shift test 7.24M
plain radiographs
   bone graft materials on 3.7M
   pathological lesions
      bone tumours 10.7–12E
      with visible fluid levels on 10.16M
   radiation dose sustained 2.10M
plantar layer of foot, third 1.18M
plates (internal fixation) 3.1–4E
   compression 8.11M
   distal radial fracture 13.16M
ploidy abnormalities 11.1M
PMMA see polymethylmethacrylate
polyethylene 8.12M
   in total joint replacement 8.21M